MCQs in Undergraduate Obstetrics and Gynaecology

Ian Johnson

BSc DM FRCOG

Professor, Department of Obstetrics and Gynaecology, University of Nottingham; Honorary Consultant Obstetrician and Gynaecologist, The City Hospital, Nottingham

Ken Dowell

MRCOG FRCS(Ed) DM

Senior Lecturer, Department of Obstetrics and Gynaecology, University of Nottingham; Honorary Consultant Obstetrician and Gynaecologist, University Hospital, Nottingham

Second Edition

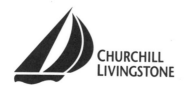

CHURCHILL LIVINGSTONE

NEW YORK EDINBURGH LONDON MADRID
MELBOURNE SAN FRANCISO AND TOKYO 1997

CHURCHILL LIVINGSTONE
An imprint of Harcourt Publishers Limited

 is a registered trademark of Harcourt Publishers Limited

First published 1985
Second edition 1994
  Reprinted 1997
  Reprinted 2000

ISBN 0 443 049599

British Library Cataloguing in Publication Data
A catalogue record for this book is available from the British Library.

Library of Congress Cataloging in Publication Data
Johnson, Ian, BSc, DM, MRCOG.
    MCQ's in undergraduate obstetrics and gynaecology/Ian Johnson,
Ken Dowell. — 2nd ed.
      p.   cm.
    Includes bibliographical references and index.
    ISBN 0-443-04959-9
    1. Obstetrics—Examinations, questions, etc. 2. Gynecology—
Examinations, questions, etc. I. Dowell, Ken. II. Title.
    [DNLM: 1. Obstetrics—examination questions. 2. Gynecology—
examination questions.   WQ 18 J67m 1994]
RG111.J64 1994
618'.076—dc20
DNLM/DLC
for Library of Congress   94-4028
                                                                        CIP

Printed in China
NPCC/03

Contents

Preface to the Second Edition

In the ten years since the first edition of this book was written multiple choice questions have continued to play a major role in the testing of factual knowledge. Undergraduate examinations have been extensively modified to include problem orientated modified essay questions, OSCEs and a reduction in the reliance on traditional essay questions. Multiple choice questions have, however, remained the most effective and objective means of assessing straightforward factual knowledge. They usually correlate far better with overall performance in examinations than any other part of the examination. Various types of multiple choice question have been introduced but we have remained with the one stem, five twig, true, false format as this is still the one that is the most commonly used in universities in the United Kingdom and is still the form in use in MRCOG Part I and Part II examinations.

The comments made in the preface to the first edition regarding the basic principles of sitting multiple choice examinations remain as true as they were in the 1980s.

I.J.
K.D.

1994

Preface to the First Edition

Multiple choice questions are, some would say unfortunately, here to stay. As a form of examination they have considerable advantages over more traditional methods. Marking is more objective and considerably faster, and a wider range of knowledge can be tested. Experience suggests that the marks achieved by students in this form of examination correlate well with their marks in other forms of written examination.

Several forms of MCQ are available, but the commonest, used throughout this book, is the single stem with five twigs, each of which may be marked true or false. Generally a single mark is awarded for a correct answer, zero for an abstention, and a penalty of one mark is deducted for each wrong answer. This form of question and marking system is the one adopted for the majority of obstetric and gynaecological undergraduate examinations and for the Royal College examinations.

Many undergraduates feel that they perform badly in MCQ examinations. In fact, this is not the case, but there is no doubt that a little forethought can make a considerable difference to the student's final mark. Firstly, there is no substitute for knowledge. Large numbers of answers are marked wrongly because of failure to read the question carefully enough. Worse still, students frequently fill in the answer form incorrectly or incompletely. Read the instructions carefully, use the correct writing instrument and fill in the correct boxes on the form. Although there is usually plenty of time to complete these examinations, it is prudent to complete the form as you go, not to leave it until having finished answering the questions in rough. Transferring large numbers of answers on to a computer form in a short time is a certain recipe for disaster.

Answering the questions in an MCQ paper is largely a matter of common sense. Although the examiner's words should usually be taken literally, the questions are not designed to stretch credulity. When the question asks if something 'may' happen, it implies that it is at least a rare or uncommon association, or even very common, not that it has never occurred before, but could do under some miraculous set of circumstances. Similarly, 'common' implies a reasonable association, but not necessarily as frequent as 'usually'.

Basic knowledge allied to common sense will deal with supposed ambiguities in most questions. Wild guessing will almost guarantee failure. It is reasonable to mark some answers when one is not absolutely sure that one is correct, but these should be calculated guesses when one is almost certain of the answer. If sufficient questions have been answered (depending on the pass mark, frequently between 50 and 60% in undergraduate examinations) there is little value in going through the paper a second time, except to spot obvious errors or misreadings of questions. It is probably more common to reduce the final mark than to improve it.

Practice MCQs have two purposes. One is to allow the student to gain experience in answering this type of question, and to avoid the pitfalls detailed above. The other, rather more important, purpose is to provide a form of self-assessment to enable the student to direct further work into the correct areas. The chapters in this book are sub-divided into major topics in obstetrics and gynaecology to make this task easier, although there is inevitably considerable overlap. A considerable portion of the book is devoted to basic sciences. Increasingly these reproductive sciences are being integrated into clinical undergraduate curricula, which is where they belong. Some of the questions are too easy, some far too difficult, but this is frequently the same as examination papers. In places there are questions in which the answer given is contentious or controversial. I hope that these do not appear too often, and that the answer given is the one most acceptable for undergraduate teaching. Discussion of most of the answers can be found in most undergraduate textbooks and a small selection of these is listed at the back of the book, together with a list of books which have also been used to compile these questions, for the more interested student.

I wish to express my thanks to Dr J. Johnson for her help in compiling and checking the manuscript and for her advice on aspects of gynaecological pathology.

1985   I.J.

1. Basic sciences

1.1 In the first half of a normal menstrual cycle

A serum progesterone levels are high
B the endometrium is rich in glycogen
C the corpus luteum begins to degenerate
D mitotic figures are seen in the endometrium
E some ovarian follicles degenerate

1.2 In the normal menstrual cycle

A mitoses occur in the menstruating endometrium
B the endometrium regenerates from the basal layer
C proliferative changes in the endometrium are caused by oestrogen and progesterone working together
D basal vacuolation is the earliest histological sign of ovulation
E endometrial cystic hyperplasia is a sign of ovulation

1.3 The endometrium

A contains many mitoses between the 6th and 10th days of the cycle
B contains large quantities of glycogen by the 10th day of the cycle
C is supplied with blood by the spiral arteries
D has long convoluted glands in the secretory phase
E is completely shed in a normal menstrual cycle

1.4 During pregnancy

A cardiac output increases by 40%
B vascular peripheral resistance increases
C heart rate increases by 25%
D stroke volume decreases by 5%
E blood pressure is unchanged

1.5 In pregnancy, the maternal

A reticulocyte count is decreased
B platelet count is increased
C neutrophil count is increased
D plasma fibrinogen concentration is increased
E plasma fibrinolytic activity is increased

(Answers overleaf)

1.1   A   **False**   In the first half of a menstrual cycle approximately
     B   **False**   20 follicles begin to mature, but usually only one
     C   **False**   will reach the stage of ovulation, the rest becoming
     D   **True**   atretic. In the second half of the cycle progesterone
     E   **True**   levels are high and the secretory endometrium
becomes rich in glycogen. The corpus luteum
begins to degenerate 12 days after ovulation unless
fertilisation has taken place.

1.2   A   **True**   At the beginning of the menstrual cycle, while
     B   **True**   menstruation is going on, the endometrium
     C   **False**   regenerates from the basal layer, cells divide and
     D   **True**   mitotic figures appear. Proliferative changes take
     E   **False**   place under the influence of oestrogen alone. Basal
vacuolation appears shortly after ovulation. Cystic
hyperplasia is an effect of oestrogen alone and
appears in anovulatory cycles.

1.3   A   **True**   The endometrium is supplied with blood via the
     B   **False**   spiral arteries. At the beginning of a cycle cell
     C   **True**   division takes place and many mitoses can be seen.
     D   **True**   After ovulation (day 14), under the combined effects
     E   **False**   of oestrogen and progesterone, the endometrial
glands become convoluted and the cells full of
glycogen. At menstruation the superficial layers are
shed.

1.4   A   **True**   During pregnancy the 40% increase in cardiac
     B   **False**   output takes place mainly in the first 16 weeks. It is
     C   **False**   mostly due to an increase in stroke volume as heart
     D   **False**   rate only increases by approximately 12%.
     E   **False**   Considerable peripheral vascular dilatation occurs,
decreasing resistance and leading to a small fall in
blood pressure in most pregnancies.

1.5   A   **False**   Although red cell count falls during pregnancy, this
     B   **False**   is because of haemodilution. There is an increase in
     C   **True**   red cell production and reticulocyte count. Platelet
     D   **True**   concentration falls slightly due to haemodilution
     E   **False**   and increased consumption. The total white cell
count rises in pregnancy due to an increase in
neutrophils. Plasma fibrinogen concentration nearly
doubles in pregnancy. Fibrinolytic activity is
decreased, possibly due to placental inhibitors.

1.6 **In normal pregnancy**
   A glomerular filtration rate increases
   B plasma urea concentration increases
   C plasma glucose concentration increases
   D plasma urate concentration falls
   E sodium reabsorption decreases

1.7 **In normal pregnancy**
   A red cell mass is increased by 15%
   B haemoglobin concentration falls
   C the total oxygen carrying capacity of the blood falls
   D plasma volume falls by 10%
   E mean corpuscular haemoglobin concentration increases

1.8 **During normal pregnancy the following decrease in blood**
   A fibrinogen concentration
   B factor VIII concentration
   C plasma renin activity
   D total calcium concentration
   E PCO_2

1.9 **In normal pregnancy**
   A plasma thyroid binding globulin concentrations increase
   B plasma thyroid stimulating hormone increases
   C plasma free thyroxine levels increase
   D iodine requirements increase
   E fetal thyroid function is independent of maternal thyroid function in the third trimester

1.10 **Concentrations of the following substances increase in maternal blood during normal pregnancy**
   A cholesterol
   B phospholipids
   C albumin
   D globulins
   E amino acids

(Answers overleaf)

1.6   A   **True**   GFR increases by approximately 40%. Nitrogenous
      B   **False**   products such as urea and uric acid are cleared
      C   **False**   from blood at a greater rate and plasma levels fall.
      D   **True**   During pregnancy sodium is retained by the kidney
      E   **False**   by increased tubular reabsorption. Fasting blood
                      glucose concentration falls slightly in pregnancy.
                      Although there is loss of glucose in the urine, the
                      change is due to factors such as hyperinsulinaemia.

1.7   A   **True**   Red cell mass increases by 15%, but plasma
      B   **True**   volume by approximately 40%. Although there is
      C   **False**   more haemoglobin present, and the oxygen
      D   **False**   carrying capacity of the blood increases, the
      E   **False**   dilutional effect causes the haemoglobin
                      concentration to fall. MCHC falls slightly.

1.8   A   **False**   Clotting factors VII, VIII and X, together with
      B   **False**   fibrinogen, all increase. Plasma renin activity
      C   **False**   increases due mainly to the increased
      D   **True**   angiotensinogen synthesis, stimulated by
      E   **True**   oestrogens. Total calcium levels are low because of
                      the reduction in albumin to bind with it. PCO_2 falls
                      because of the increase in respiratory function.

1.9   A   **True**   Iodine requirements in pregnancy increase because
      B   **False**   of increased iodide excretion in the urine and
      C   **False**   placental trapping of iodine. Raised thyroid binding
      D   **True**   globulin concentration is due to oestrogen
      E   **True**   stimulation of its synthesis. Total thyroxine levels
                      consequently increase, but free thyroxine does not.
                      In the second half of pregnancy maternal T_4, T_3 and
                      TSH will not cross the placenta and fetal thyroid
                      function is autonomous.

1.10 A   **True**   Lipids increase in plasma during pregnancy. Total
      B   **True**   protein concentration falls, mainly due to the
      C   **False**   decrease in albumin, but globulins show a small
      D   **True**   increase. The changes in concentrations of some of
      E   **False**   the globulins, particularly binding proteins, are of
                      importance in pregnancy. Total amino acid
                      concentration falls, although there are wide
                      variations between individual amino acids.

1.11 In the gastrointestinal tract in pregnancy

A stomach motility is decreased
B stomach acid production increases
C transit time of food in the small intestine is increased
D folate absorption is increased
E iron absorption is increased

1.12 In the renal tract in pregnancy

A the renal pelvic calyces are dilated
B the ureters are dilated
C the left side is more affected than the right
D bladder tone increases
E multigravidae show greater changes than primigravidae

1.13 During pregnancy, in patients not taking iron supplements

A serum iron concentration decreases
B total iron binding capacity is a reliable indicator of the state of iron stores
C plasma transferrin concentration increases
D plasma ferritin concentration decreases
E fetal iron stores are not affected by maternal iron store state

1.14 The following respiratory volumes and functions increase during pregnancy

A expiratory reserve volume
B tidal volume
C respiratory rate
D residual volume
E inspiratory reserve

(Answers overleaf)

1.11 A **True**   Stomach acid and pepsin secretion are reduced in
     B **False**   pregnancy. Generalised relaxation of smooth
     C **True**   muscle leads to a lack of tone in the stomach with
     D **False**   reduced motility and increased transit time of food
     E **True**   in the small intestine. Despite the increased transit
                   time there is little evidence for increased absorption
                   of foodstuffs. Folate absorption is either unaltered
                   or slightly decreased. Iron absorption increases, but
                   this probably represents a normal response to
                   decreased serum iron.

1.12 A **True**   In pregnancy the renal tract is dilated. This may be
     B **True**   due to the effect of progesterone in relaxing
     C **False**   smooth muscle, but because the right side is
     D **False**   affected more than the left and the uterus is more
     E **False**   often dextro-rotated it may be due to pressure of
                   the gravid uterus on the ureters at the pelvic brim.
                   Bladder tone is unaltered. Primigravidae are more
                   affected than multigravidae.

1.13 A **True**   The increased requirement for iron during
     B **False**   pregnancy is not met from diet alone in most
     C **True**   women. Consequently, serum iron concentration
     D **True**   falls and there is an increase in iron binding
     E **False**   capacity as the β_1 globulin transferrin concentration
                   rises. Iron binding capacity and serum iron
                   measurements fluctuate widely and do not
                   accurately reflect iron status. Ferritin is far more
                   stable and does reflect iron stores. There is a rapid
                   fall in plasma ferritin concentration in early
                   pregnancy. Fetal plasma ferritin concentration is
                   greater than maternal, but reflects the maternal
                   status.

1.14 A **False**   Expiratory reserve volume falls progressively from
     B **True**   early pregnancy, from approximately 1300 ml to
     C **False**   1100 ml by term. Tidal volume rises throughout
     D **False**   pregnancy, to a total increase of approximately
     E **True**   40%. The respiratory rate is unchanged. The
                   residual volume falls by approximately 20%.
                   Inspiratory reserve increases progressively
                   throughout pregnancy.

1.15 During normal pregnancy, maternal

A   plasma parathyroid hormone concentration increases
B   calcium absorption increases
C   plasma calcium concentration increases
D   parathyroid hormone crosses the placenta to the fetus
E   plasma calcium concentration is less than fetal plasma calcium concentration

1.16 In the fetus at term

A   haemoglobin has a higher affinity for oxygen than in the adult
B   there is no adult haemoglobin
C   erythropoiesis is mainly hepatic
D   the haemoglobin concentration is greater than in the adult
E   haemoglobin is more resistant to acid denaturation than adult haemoglobin

1.17 At birth

A   pressure in the right side of the heart increases
B   the foramen ovale closes immediately
C   pulmonary vascular resistance falls
D   increased arterial oxygen tension causes closure of the ductus arteriosus
E   increased prostaglandin release causes closure of the ductus arteriosus

1.18 Transfer of oxygen from the mother to the fetus is promoted by

A   active transport
B   the higher affinity of fetal than maternal haemoglobin for oxygen
C   the fetal to maternal haemoglobin concentration ratio
D   the high placental pool PO_2 when compared with alveolar PO_2
E   the concentration gradient between quantities of oxygen carried in maternal and fetal blood

1.19 In the early stages of hypoxia in the fetus

A   systemic vasodilatation occurs
B   vessels in the cerebral circulation dilate
C   cardiac output increases
D   bradycardia occurs
E   cerebral tissue oxygen concentration is normal

(Answers overleaf)

1.15 A **True**   During pregnancy calcium requirements increase,
     B **True**   mainly for the fetal skeleton. Maternal parathyroid
     C **False** hormone secretion is increased, which leads to
     D **False** increased absorption of calcium from the gut.
     E **True**   However, total plasma calcium concentration
                  decreases, mainly due to haemodilution. Calcium is
                  actively transported into the fetus, which has a
                  higher plasma calcium concentration than the
                  mother. The fetus controls its own calcium
                  metabolism, neither parathyroid hormone nor
                  calcitonin crossing the placenta from the mother.

1.16 A **True**   Haemoglobin F (HbF) has a higher affinity for
     B **False** oxygen than adult haemoglobin. It co-exists with
     C **False** adult haemoglobin at birth and is gradually
     D **True**   replaced by it in the first year of life. The resistance
     E **True**   of HbF to acid or alkali denaturation is the basis of
                  the Kleihauer test. Erythropoiesis is mainly hepatic
                  in the second trimester of pregnancy. The
                  haemoglobin concentration at birth is usually
                  approximately 17 g/dl.

1.17 A **False** When the umbilical vessels are occluded there is a
     B **False** decreased venous return, lowering the pressure in
     C **True**   the right side of the heart. The foramen ovale
     D **True**   gradually closes. Pressure in the pulmonary
     E **False** vasculature falls as the first breath is taken. The
                  ductus arteriosus is sensitive to arterial oxygen
                  tension, an increase causing it to close.
                  Prostaglandin synthetase inhibitors, such as aspirin
                  or indomethacin, may also cause closure
                  prematurely in some cases when these drugs are
                  given in pregnancy in sufficient dose.

1.18 A **False** Oxygen passes from the mother to the fetus by
     B **True**   simple diffusion. Fetal blood contains
     C **True**   approximately 60% more oxygen per 100 ml than
     D **False** does maternal, despite the placental pool PO_2 being
     E **False** only 30% that of alveolar PO_2. This is because of
                  the high affinity of haemoglobin F for oxygen and
                  the high fetal haemoglobin concentration.

1.19 A **False** Blood flow to the fetal brain is regulated in an
     B **True**   attempt to maintain the tissue oxygen
     C **True**   concentration. In mild hypoxia there is an increased
     D **False** sympathetic stimulation which causes tachycardia
     E **True**   and increases cardiac output. Cerebral bloodflow is
                  maintained by a combination of dilatation of
                  cerebral vessels and constriction of some systemic
                  vessel beds.

1.20 Factors directly affecting birthweight include

    A maternal weight
    B paternal height
    C maternal age
    D birth order
    E gender

1.21 Surfactant

    A first appears in amniotic fluid after 36 weeks
    B is synthesised from sphingomyelin
    C contains lecithin
    D decreases the surface tension of the pulmonary alveoli
    E is a steroid

1.22 Amniotic fluid

    A alphafetoprotein concentration increases to term
    B bilirubin concentration increases to 36 weeks gestation
    C is hyperosmolar to fetal plasma
    D is mainly formed from fetal urine
    E urea concentration increases to term

1.23 Amniotic fluid

    A first appears at seven weeks gestation
    B reaches a maximum volume at 38 weeks
    C in early pregnancy has a composition similar to maternal plasma
    D passes through fetal skin up to 36 weeks gestation
    E has an acid pH

1.24 Prostaglandins

    A are small peptides
    B are synthesised by vascular endothelium
    C are stored in granules
    D are metabolised in platelets
    E have a half life of one hour in plasma

1.25 Progesterone

    A relaxes the myometrium
    B stimulates respiration
    C is given orally for therapeutic purposes
    D causes a fall in basal body temperature
    E is a glycoprotein

(Answers overleaf)

1.20 A **True** The single most important determinant of
     B **True** birthweight is gestation but other maternal and
     C **False** paternal factors will also modify an individual's
     D **True** potential birthweight. The most important of these
     E **True** is maternal weight followed by paternal height and
             gender. The birth order is important in that first
             babies are significantly lighter than subsequent
             ones although after the first pregnancy differences
             tend to be small. Maternal age is unimportant when
             other factors are taken into account.

1.21 A **False** Surfactant appears in amniotic fluid in large
     B **False** quantities before 34 weeks gestation and can be
     C **True** detected much earlier. It is made up mainly of
     D **True** phospholipid, particularly lecithin, and is not
     E **False** synthesised from sphyngomyelin. Its function is to
             decrease surface tension in pulmonary alveoli and
             prevent their collapse.

1.22 A **False** Alphafetoprotein concentration is maximal at
     B **False** 13 weeks and bilirubin at approximately 24 weeks.
     C **False** The amniotic fluid is mainly formed from fetal
     D **True** urine, and reflects the maturing fetal kidney,
     E **True** becoming progressively more hypo-osmolar and
             containing increasing concentrations of nitrogenous
             products such as urea.

1.23 A **False** Amniotic fluid appears seven days after fertilisation
     B **True** and reaches a maximum volume at 38 weeks. In
     C **True** early pregnancy the composition is similar to that
     D **False** of maternal plasma but as the fetal kidney matures
     E **False** it becomes more like fetal urine. The pH is always
             greater than seven. Fetal skin is permeable until
             keratinisation takes place at 24 weeks.

1.24 A **False** Prostaglandins are 20 carbon derivatives of
     B **True** prostanoic acid. They are synthesised in vascular
     C **False** endothelium as required and are not stored, being
     D **True** rapidly metabolised, particularly in lungs and
     E **False** platelets.

1.25 A **True** Progesterone is a steroid hormone that is produced
     B **True** mainly by the corpus luteum and placenta. It is not
     C **False** active when given orally. In ovulatory menstrual
     D **False** cycles it is the cause of the rise in basal body
     E **False** temperature in the second half of the cycle. In
             pregnancy it relaxes smooth muscle, including the
             myometrium, and stimulates respiration.

1.26 **Prolactin**
A   secretion is promoted by dopamine
B   release is stimulated by oestradiol
C   release is stimulated by thyrotropin releasing factor
D   plasma concentrations increase in pregnancy
E   is responsible for milk ejection

1.27 **Human chorionic gonadotrophin**
A   is produced by the pre-implantation blastocyst
B   is a steroid hormone
C   reaches its maximum concentration in maternal plasma at 20 weeks gestation
D   is mainly produced by the corpus luteum
E   maintains the corpus luteum in early pregnancy

1.28 **In the human testis**
A   oestrogens are formed
B   testosterone concentration is the same as in the plasma
C   arterial blood is cooler than venous blood
D   most of the androgen content is dihydrotestosterone
E   androstenedione is secreted

1.29 **The Sertoli cells of the testis**
A   have FSH receptors
B   are directly stimulated by luteinising hormone
C   produce testosterone
D   produce inhibin
E   secrete prolactin

1.30 **Dihydrotestosterone**
A   is a less potent androgen than testosterone
B   is responsible for the development of the male external genitalia
C   is a precursor of testosterone
D   is responsible for male pattern baldness
E   is produced from oestrone in adipose tissue

1.31 **Luteinising hormone**
A   plasma concentration is increased in pregnancy
B   stimulates androgen production
C   plasma concentrations are increased in girls with Turner's syndrome
D   is a steroid hormone
E   is released at a constant rate throughout the ovulatory menstrual cycle

(Answers overleaf)

1.26 A **False** Dopamine inhibits prolactin release from the
B **True** anterior pituitary. Release is stimulated by
C **True** oestradiol and TRF. In pregnancy, because of high
D **True** oestrogen levels, prolactin concentration in plasma
E **False** is high. Milk ejection, contraction of the
myoepithelial cells in the breast, is due to
stimulation by oxytocin.

1.27 A **True** HCG is produced by the pre-implantation blastocyst
B **False** and later by the developed trophoblast. It is a
C **False** glycoprotein which reaches a maximal level at
D **False** 70 days gestation. One of its actions is to maintain
E **True** the corpus luteum until the placenta takes over
steroid hormone production.

1.28 A **True** Steroidogenic tissue in the testis produces many
B **False** steroid hormones, including oestrogens and
C **False** androstenedione, although mostly testosterone,
D **False** which reaches a concentration 100 times that of
E **True** plasma. Testosterone is converted into
dihydrotestosterone in the target tissues, not the
testis. Arterial blood enters the scrotum and cools,
so venous blood has a lower temperature than
arterial.

1.29 A **True** Sertoli cells have FSH and testosterone receptors
B **False** and produce inhibin which controls FSH release. LH
C **False** stimulates Leydig cells to produce testosterone.
D **True** Prolactin is not produced by the testis.
E **False**

1.30 A **False** Testosterone is converted in target tissues to its
B **True** more potent metabolite dihydrotestosterone. It is
C **False** this substance that is responsible for the
D **True** development of male external genitalia and
E **False** secondary sexual characteristics. In the absence of
conversion, even with normal testes, the individual
is phenotypically female (testicular feminisation
syndrome). Androstenedione converts to oestrone
in adipose tissue.

1.31 A **False** Luteinising hormone acts on Leydig cells in the
B **True** male to stimulate testosterone secretion and
C **True** release. In Turner's syndrome there is primary
D **False** gonadal failure and the hypothalamic/pituitary
E **False** response is to release FSH and LH. Luteinising
hormone is a glycoprotein that is released at
relatively low levels in pregnancy and in the
menstrual cycle except for the mid-cycle peak
before ovulation.

1.32 Follicle stimulating hormone
A stimulates spermatogenesis
B plasma concentration is high in Klinefelter syndrome
C is produced in the hypothalamus
D stimulates ovarian oestrogen production
E prevents regression of the corpus luteum

1.33 Human decidua produces
A prostaglandin $F_2\alpha$
B prostaglandin E_2
C alphafetoprotein
D progesterone
E human chorionic gonadotrophin

1.34 During lactation
A oestrogens promote milk release
B the suckling reflex increases oxytocin release
C the suckling reflex increases prolactin release
D ovulation is reliably suppressed
E human placental lactogen is required for milk synthesis

1.35 Oestrogen
A is produced in the corpus luteum
B cannot be detected in the blood of postmenopausal women
C is mainly secreted by the ovary as oestrone
D is responsible for secretory changes in the endometrium
E is the dominant gonadal hormone at puberty

1.36 Oestrogens
A are responsible for the initial growth of the breast at puberty
B stimulate sebaceous gland activity
C reduce FSH release from the pituitary
D stimulate inhibin production in the testis
E stimulate release of prolactin from the pituitary

(Answers overleaf)

1.32 A **True**   Follicle stimulating hormone is produced in the
      B **True**   anterior pituitary. In the male it acts on the Sertoli
      C **False** cells and promotes spermatogenesis. In the female
      D **True**   it stimulates follicles and promotes oestrogen
      E **False** production. It has no effect on the corpus luteum.
                    Klinefelter syndrome produces a primary testicular
                    failure and the hypothalamic/pituitary response is to
                    release FSH and LH in high concentration.

1.33 A **True**   Endometrium and decidua both produce
      B **True**   prostaglandins $F_2\alpha$ and E_2. Alphafetoprotein and
      C **False** human chorionic gonadotrophin come from the
      D **False** fetus and placenta and some ovarian tumours, but
      E **False** not the uterus. Decidua does not produce steroid
                    hormones.

1.34 A **False** During lactation the suckling reflex promotes milk
      B **True**   synthesis by causing a release of prolactin and milk
      C **True**   ejection by causing a release of oxytocin.
      D **False** Oestrogens increase prolactin secretion, but high
      E **False** concentrations block some of the effects of
                    prolactin in the breast and suppress lactation.
                    Ovulation is suppressed by the raised prolactin, but
                    not reliably. HPL is a placental hormone and is no
                    longer present during lactation.

1.35 A **True**   The corpus luteum produces both oestrogens and
      B **False** progesterone and most of the ovarian oestrogens
      C **False** are in the form of oestradiol. Oestrogens are
      D **False** responsible for proliferative changes in
      E **True**   endometrium. At puberty the first few cycles are
                    anovulatory and consequently oestrogen acts
                    without progesterone. After the menopause
                    oestrone is formed from androstenedione secreted
                    by the adrenals.

1.36 A **True**   Anovulatory cycles at puberty cause oestrogens to
      B **False** work alone and cause the initial breast growth.
      C **True**   Androgens stimulate sebaceous gland activity.
      D **False** Oestrogens inhibit FSH release. Inhibin release is
      E **True**   stimulated by FSH. Oestrogens interfere with
                    dopaminergic inhibition of prolactin release and
                    thus cause secretion of prolactin.

1.37 Oxytocin is
A   synthesised in the anterior hypothalamic nuclei
B   an antidiuretic
C   stored in the anterior pituitary
D   a polypeptide hormone
E   important as a cause of uterine contractions in early pregnancy

1.38 After the menopause
A   FSH levels fall
B   luteinising hormone levels fall
C   plasma progesterone concentration increases
D   ovarian oestrogen production ceases
E   plasma prolactin concentration falls

1.39 Puberty in the female
A   breast development usually begins before the appearance of pubic hair
B   the ovaries are not sensitive to gonadotrophins before puberty
C   increased production of adrenal androgens precedes puberty
D   before puberty plasma FSH concentrations are high
E   the first few menstrual cycles are normally anovulatory

1.40 The lower segment of the uterus
A   develops in the first trimester
B   contains no muscle fibres
C   lies below the uterovesical fold of peritoneum
D   is less vascular than the upper segment
E   is lined by squamous epithelium

1.41 The major supports of the uterus are
A   the transverse cervical (cardinal) ligaments
B   the infundibulo-pelvic ligament
C   the round ligaments
D   the uterosacral ligaments
E   the pubo-cervical ligaments

(Answers overleaf)

1.37 A **True**   Oxytocin is synthesised in the paraventricular
      B **True**   nucleus of the hypothalamus, transported along
      C **False**   nerve trunks and stored in the posterior pituitary. It
      D **True**   is a small peptide, very similar in structure to
      E **False**   antidiuretic hormone with some overlap in effect.
                     The action of oxytocin on the uterus depends upon
                     oestrogen priming and is relatively weak in early
                     pregnancy.

1.38 A **False**   After the menopause there is primary ovarian
      B **False**   failure. Follicles no longer develop and the
      C **False**   oestradiol production falls, although some
      D **False**   oestrogens are still produced. FSH and LH levels
      E **True**   are released from control and increase. No corpora
                     lutea form and progesterone levels are low.
                     Prolactin concentration usually mirrors oestrogen
                     concentration, and consequently is low.

1.39 A **True**   Before puberty the hypothalamus is very sensitive
      B **False**   to oestrogens. In a process involving an increase in
      C **True**   the production of adrenal androgens, this sensitivity
      D **False**   is re-aligned to allow release of firstly FSH and then
      E **True**   LH, both of which are at low levels before puberty.
                     The ovarian sensitivity to gonadotrophins is
                     unchanged. The sequence of events in puberty
                     usually involves breast development, followed by
                     the appearance of body hair and finally
                     menstruation. After menstruation the first few
                     cycles are usually anovulatory.

1.40 A **False**   The lower segment of the uterus is derived from
      B **False**   the isthmus and lies below the point at which the
      C **True**   uterovesical fold of peritoneum reflects. It develops
      D **True**   late in the third trimester of pregnancy and consists
      E **False**   of muscle and fibrous tissue, mainly the latter. It is
                     less vascular than the upper segment, but is lined
                     by thin decidualised endometrium.

1.41 A **True**   The pelvic ligaments that support the uterus are the
      B **False**   pubo-cervical anteriorly, the uterosacrals postero-
      C **False**   laterally and the cardinals laterally. These ligaments
      D **True**   are important in the prevention of uterovaginal
      E **True**   prolapse. The round ligaments have a very minor
                     role, if any, in supporting the uterus. The
                     infundibulo-pelvic ligament is a fold of peritoneum
                     running from the outer aspect of the broad
                     ligament to the pelvic side wall. It contains the
                     ovarian vessels.

1.42 **In the female pelvis, the ureter**
  A   is derived from the urogenital sinus
  B   runs over the uterine artery
  C   crosses the bifurcation of the common iliac artery
  D   runs within the broad ligament
  E   enters the bladder on its anterior aspect

1.43 **The female urinary bladder**
  A   is separated from the symphysis pubis by a fold of
       peritoneum
  B   is joined to the umbilicus by the urachus
  C   is supplied by the inferior epigastric artery
  D   has a muscle coat continuous with that of the urethra
  E   receives innervation from the pudendal nerve

1.44 **Arteries supplying the ureter include**
  A   inferior vesical
  B   ovarian
  C   inferior epigastric
  D   external iliac
  E   uterine

1.45 **The right ovarian artery**
  A   is a branch of the right renal artery
  B   runs in the infundibulo-pelvic fold
  C   runs posterior to the inferior vena cava
  D   supplies branches to the third part of the duodenum
  E   anastomoses with the right uterine artery

1.46 **The pudendal nerve**
  A   leaves the pelvis through the lesser sciatic foramen
  B   innervates the internal sphincter of the rectum
  C   supplies the levator ani
  D   lies on the supra-spinous ligament
  E   has the perineal nerve as its terminal branch

1.47 **The nerve supply of the vulva and perineum is derived from
       the following nerves**
  A   pudendal
  B   genito-femoral
  C   obturator
  D   anterior cutaneous of thigh
  E   posterior cutaneous of thigh

(Answers overleaf)

1.42 A **False** The ureter develops from the ureteric bud, an
      B **False** outgrowth of the caudal part of the mesonephric
      C **True**   duct. It runs across the bifurcation of the common
      D **True**   iliac artery, within the broad ligament and under the
      E **False** uterine artery, entering the bladder at the lateral
                    point of the trigone.

1.43 A **False** The bladder is anteriorly in direct relation to the
      B **True**   symphysis pubis, the peritoneum reflects from the
      C **True**   fundus of the bladder to the uterus. Innervation of
      D **True**   the bladder is from the hypogastric nerves. The
      E **False** pudendal nerve supplies the urethra.

1.44 A **True**   The ureter takes its blood supply from a variety of
      B **True**   sources as it passes through the abdomen and
      C **False** pelvis. In the pelvis it relates to the internal iliac
      D **False** system rather than the external iliac.
      E **True**

1.45 A **False** The right ovarian artery arises directly from the
      B **True**   aorta below the origin of the renal arteries. It runs
      C **False** anterior to the inferior vena cava and does not have
      D **False** any intra-abdominal branches. It runs in the
      E **True**   infundibulo-pelvic fold of the peritoneum and
                    eventually anastomoses with the right uterine artery.

1.46 A **False** The pudendal nerve leaves the pelvis through the
      B **False** greater sciatic foramen and enters the perineum
      C **True**   through the lesser sciatic foramen. It supplies the
      D **True**   external sphincter of the rectum together with the
      E **True**   levator ani.

1.47 A **True**   The pudendal nerve innervates most of the
      B **True**   perineum and vulva. Further sensory branches to
      C **False** the skin are derived from the pudendal branch of
      D **False** the posterior cutaneous nerve of the thigh and the
      E **True**   femoral branch of the genito-femoral nerve.

1.48 The vulval blood supply is via the
- A   internal pudendal artery
- B   external pudendal artery
- C   superior vesical artery
- D   middle rectal artery
- E   vaginal artery

1.49 Lymphatic drainage of the body of the uterus is to the following nodes
- A   sacral
- B   superficial inguinal
- C   obturator
- D   femoral
- E   external iliac

1.50 The cervix
- A   is made up mainly of smooth muscle
- B   is made up mainly of voluntary muscle
- C   is covered with peritoneum anteriorly
- D   has pain sensation to pelvic splanchnic nerves
- E   lies 1 cm medial to both ureters

1.51 The vagina
- A   contains mucus secreting glands
- B   relates posteriorly to the rectum in its middle third
- C   relates anteriorly to the bladder base in its lowest third
- D   is supplied in part by the uterine artery
- E   is entirely derived from the paramesonephric duct

1.52 The ampulla of the fallopian tube
- A   is derived from the paramesonephric duct
- B   obtains its blood supply partly from the ovarian artery
- C   has a lymphatic drainage to the para-aortic nodes
- D   has a complex folding of its mucosa
- E   has an external circular muscle coat

(Answers overleaf)

1.48   A   **True**   The vulva is a very vascular area, supplied by
      B   **True**   branches of the internal pudendal arteries from the
      C   **False**   internal iliac artery and the external pudendal
      D   **False**   arteries from the femoral arteries.
      E   **False**

1.49   A   **True**   The lymphatic drainage of the body of the uterus is
      B   **True**   mainly to the external and internal iliac nodes, with
      C   **True**   some drainage to sacral and obturator nodes. A
      D   **False**   small amount follows the round ligaments from the
      E   **True**   fundus of the uterus to the inguinal canals and the
                        inguinal nodes.

1.50   A   **False**   The cervix consists mainly of connective tissue. The
      B   **False**   peritoneum reflects from the uterus over the
      C   **False**   bladder above the level of the internal os. The
      D   **True**   ureters lie in the base of the broad ligaments
      E   **True**   approximately 1 cm lateral to the cervix on each
                        side.

1.51   A   **False**   The vagina contains no glands. Apparent discharge
      B   **True**   is uterine or cervical, transudation and
      C   **False**   desquamation from the vaginal epithelium, or
      D   **True**   ascending from Bartholin's glands. Posteriorly it is
      E   **False**   related, from above down, to the pouch of Douglas,
                        the rectum and the perineal body. Anteriorly from
                        above down, it relates to the bladder and, in its
                        lowest third, the urethra. The vaginal blood supply
                        is mainly from the vaginal artery, but in the upper
                        part some supply is from the uterine artery, which
                        anastomoses with the vaginal. The vagina forms
                        from a downgrowth of the Mullerian duct and an
                        upgrowth of the urogenital sinus which together
                        form the vaginal plate.

1.52   A   **True**   The fallopian tube is entirely derived from the
      B   **True**   paramesonephric ducts. The blood supply of the
      C   **True**   ampulla is mainly from the ovarian artery, and
      D   **True**   lymphatic drainage, as with the ovary, is directly to
      E   **False**   the para-aortic nodes. The ampulla contains a
                        mucous membrane that is folded in a very complex
                        manner, increasingly so as the fimbriae are
                        approached. There is an inner circular and an outer
                        longitudinal muscle coat.

1.53 The ovary

A   is derived from the paramesonephros
B   is attached to the uterine cornu by the infundibulo-pelvic
     ligament
C   lies posterior to the broad ligament
D   lies anterior to the ureter
E   is attached to the distal portion of the fallopian tube

1.54 In the fetal circulation

A   the ductus arteriosus carries blood to the lungs
B   there is one umbilical vein
C   oxygenated blood passes through the foramen ovale
D   the ductus venosus carries blood with a lower PO_2 than
     umbilical arterial blood
E   the ductus arteriosus closes during the last four weeks of
     pregnancy

1.55 In spermatogenesis

A   the Leydig cells are mainly responsible for sperm
     production
B   spermatids are haploid
C   new sperms develop and mature in 40 days
D   spermatogonia constantly divide by mitosis
E   capacitation in the epididymis is an essential step

1.56 In the female the urogenital sinus gives rise to

A   the urethra
B   Bartholin's glands
C   the cervix
D   the trigone of the bladder
E   Gartner's duct

1.57 The fetal testes

A   secrete testosterone
B   are necessary for the formation of the mesonephric
     (Wolffian) ducts
C   produce Mullerian inhibitory factor
D   are distinguishable from fetal ovaries 30 days after
     fertilisation
E   contain cells that have migrated from the yolk sac

(Answers overleaf)

1.53 A **False** The ovary is derived from the genital ridge and
       B **False** primordial germ cells from the yolk sac. It is not a
       C **True**   Mullerian structure. The ovary is attached to the
       D **True**   pelvic side wall by the infundibulo-pelvic ligament
       E **False** which contains its blood vessels, and to the uterine
                cornu by the ovarian suspensory ligament. It lies
                posterior to the broad ligament and is anterior to
                the ureter. There is no connection to the fallopian
                tube.

1.54 A **False** The ductus arteriosus carries blood from the
       B **True**   pulmonary artery to the aorta (i.e. bypassing the
       C **True**   lungs). If it closed during pregnancy the infant
       D **False** would develop pulmonary hypertension; it closes
       E **False** after delivery. The single umbilical vein (two
                arteries) carries oxygenated blood from the
                placenta to the ductus venosus and portal veins,
                through the inferior vena cava to the right atrium,
                directly through the foramen ovale to the left atrium.

1.55 A **False** Unlike the female in whom all germ cells are
       B **True**   present in the ovary at birth, in the male
       C **False** spermatogonia constantly divide to form new germ
       D **True**   cells. These are mitotic divisions, the meiotic
       E **False** division occurring later to yield haploid spermatids.
                The process of spermatogenesis takes
                approximately 70 days and is mainly under the
                control of the Sertoli cells. Capacitation in the
                epididymis is no longer thought to be a necessary
                step; sperm obtained before this phase have been
                shown to be capable of fertilising an ovum.

1.56 A **True**   The urogenital sinus gives rise to the structures of
       B **True**   the vulva, urethra and most of the bladder. The
       C **False** trigone of the bladder is formed from the distal
       D **False** portion of the ureteric buds as the ureters are
       E **False** absorbed into the bladder. The cervix is a Mullerian
                structure. Gartner's duct is the remnant of the
                Wolffian duct in the female.

1.57 A **True**   Germ cells originate beneath the epithelium of the
       B **False** yolk sac and migrate to the genital ridge. In the
       C **True**   male the testis is identifiable from seven weeks
       D **False** after fertilisation. Testosterone is produced which
       E **True**   sustains rather than causes formation of the
                Wolffian ducts, which also appear in females.
                Mullerian inhibitory factor is produced which
                prevents development of the fallopian tubes, uterus
                and vagina.

1.58 After fertilisation

    A   cell divisions are mitotic
    B   divisions are synchronous
    C   the first division takes place within 16 hours
    D   passage down the fallopian tube takes about four days
    E   the second polar body is excluded

1.59 In the female fetus primordial germ cells

    A   differentiate by seven weeks after conception
    B   undergo the first meiotic division in the yolk sac
    C   undergo the second meiotic division in the ovarian cortex
    D   progressively decrease in number after birth
    E   are responsible for the regression of the Wolffian system

1.60 The placenta

    A   has approximately 20 cotyledons
    B   develops mainly from cytotrophoblast
    C   is covered on the maternal surface by chorion
    D   is a major endocrine organ
    E   has reached its definitive form by the fourth month of gestation

1.61 Trophoblast

    A   enters the maternal circulation
    B   is genetically maternal
    C   causes decidualisation of endometrium
    D   growth is influenced more by paternal than maternal chromosomes
    E   produces proteolytic enzymes

1.62 Early haematogenous spread is a characteristic of

    A   ovarian epithelial cancers
    B   choriocarcinoma
    C   endometrial cancer
    D   malignant melanoma of the vulva
    E   squamous cancer of the cervix

(Answers overleaf)

1.58 A **True**   The meiotic division of the female germ cell begins
      B **False** in utero, is completed after fertilisation by extrusion
      C **False** of the second polar body (2nd or mitotic division).
      D **True**   All subsequent divisions are mitotic. Divisions are
      E **True**   asynchronous and the first division takes place
                    approximately 30 hours after fertilisation.

1.59 A **False** Primordial germ cells differentiate into oogonia at
      B **False** 12 weeks after conception. The first meiotic
      C **False** (reduction) division takes place in the ovarian
      D **True**   cortex and arrests at this stage. Just before
      E **False** ovulation the first division is completed and the
                    second begins, being completed after fertilisation.
                    The Wolffian system regresses in the absence of
                    testosterone.

1.60 A **True**   In the week old ovum the trophoblast forms two
      B **True**   layers. It is clear that the syncitiotrophoblast is
      C **False** derived from the cytotrophoblast. By the fourth
      D **True**   week of life the placenta is a vascularised villous
      E **True**   organ. Villi orientated towards the uterine cavity
                    degenerate to form the chorion laeve. Those
                    remaining grow rapidly (chorion frondosum). Septa
                    appear in the third month, dividing the placenta
                    into 15–20 cotyledons. By the fourth month the
                    placenta has reached its definitive structure. Growth
                    continues, but no alteration in architecture. The
                    maternal surface is the decidual-trophoblastic
                    interface.

1.61 A **True**   Trophoblast invades decidua (endometrium
      B **False** decidualised by oestrogens and progesterone)
      C **False** producing proteolytic enzymes that enable
      D **True**   trophoblastic cells to penetrate maternal vascular
      E **True**   space. It is genetically fetal, but influenced more by
                    the paternal genetic contribution; in hydatidiform
                    mole, a gross over-growth of trophoblast with no
                    fetus present, the entire genetic complement is
                    derived from the father.

1.62 A **False** Ovarian epithelial tumours spread transcoelomically
      B **True**   in the first instance. Endothelial and cervical
      C **False** cancers spread locally and then via lymphatics. In
      D **True**   all three of these cases haematogenous spread is
      E **False** late. Although squamous cancer of the vulva
                    spreads locally and via lymphatics, the much less
                    common malignant melanoma spread via the blood
                    at an early stage.

1.63 Intraepithelial neoplasia is characterised by
  A   increased epithelial thickness
  B   increased mitotic activity
  C   breaching of the basement membrane
  D   loss of polarity
  E   increased nuclear cytoplasmic ratio

1.64 The effects of ionising radiation
  A   may take six weeks to occur
  B   are greater in well oxygenated tissues
  C   are greatest in slow growing cells
  D   include chromosomal non-disjunction
  E   include fibrosis within two weeks

1.65 In diagnostic imaging, ultrasound
  A   penetrates tissues better at low frequency
  B   at high frequency has improved resolution
  C   energy is pulsed
  D   provides measurements accurate to 0.1 mm
  E   causes acceleration of cell division

1.66 IgM immunoglobulins
  A   cross the placenta
  B   are the antibodies involved in rhesus disease
  C   are produced by the fetus
  D   are the ABO blood group antibodies
  E   are involved in the primary response to infection

1.67 A woman who is genotypically cde cde (Rhesus blood group)
  A   will have children who will all be Rhesus negative
  B   will have anti-D in her plasma
  C   is Rhesus negative
  D   is at risk of Rhesus iso-immunisation
  E   should be given an anti-D injection after each pregnancy

(Answers overleaf)

1.63	A	**False**	Intraepithelial neoplasia is potentially a
	B	**True**	premalignant condition in squamous epithelium. It
	C	**False**	is characterised by failure of maturation of the
	D	**True**	epithelium leading to loss of polarity, large nuclei
	E	**True**	and, in severe forms, many mitoses. The epithelium

is not necessarily thickened. Breaching the basement membrane is a feature of invasive cancer (i.e. not intraepithelial).

1.64	A	**True**	After exposure to ionising radiation, effects such as
	B	**True**	fibrosis take many weeks to appear. The effects of
	C	**False**	radiation are greatest in rapidly dividing cells, such
	D	**True**	as gut epithelium or tumours.
	E	**False**	

1.65	A	**True**	Ultrasound at intensities used for diagnostic
	B	**True**	imaging has no effect on cell division. Accuracy to
	C	**True**	within 1 mm is to be expected.
	D	**False**	
	E	**False**	

1.66	A	**False**	IgM immunoglobulins are too large to cross the
	B	**False**	placenta. They are responsible for the primary
	C	**True**	response to infection in mother and fetus. Anti-B
	D	**True**	and anti-A are IgM, but Rhesus antibodies are IgG
	E	**True**	(and do cross the placenta).

1.67	A	**False**	The genotype cde cde is the commonest found in
	B	**False**	Rhesus negative people. The state of being Rhesus
	C	**True**	positive or negative is determined by the D antigen;
	D	**True**	those that have it are positive. A Rhesus negative
	E	**False**	woman will not have anti-D in her plasma unless

she has been iso-immunised. She is at risk of iso-immunisation if fetal blood passes into her circulation, particularly at delivery. However, if the fetus is itself Rhesus negative there is no risk and she does not require an injection of anti-D after delivery. In this case, whether or not the infant would be Rhesus negative depends on the father's genotype; D is dominant.

1.68 In diseases inherited via dominant genes
  A   both parents must have the gene for it to be expressed
  B   penetrance is often variable
  C   at least one grandparent must have the gene
  D   siblings of an affected individual have a 1 in 4 chance of
       having the gene
  E   normal children of affected parents have normal offspring

1.69 X-linked inherited disorders include
  A   adrenogenital syndrome
  B   phenylketonuria
  C   achondroplasia
  D   glucose-6-phosphate dehydrogenase deficiency
  E   Turner's syndrome

1.70 In Down syndrome
  A   maternal karyotype is usually abnormal
  B   paternal karyotype is usually abnormal
  C   the abnormality has usually been caused by non-
       disjunction during meiosis
  D   the chromosome number is normal (46) in approximately
       5% of cases
  E   the patient is triploid in most cases

1.71 If a man has haemophilia
  A   all of his brothers will have the disease
  B   his sisters have a 1 in 2 chance of being carriers
  C   none of his sons will be affected
  D   all of his daughters will be carriers
  E   his father will have had the disease

1.72 The following drugs have tocolytic activity
  A   magnesium sulphate
  B   nifedipine
  C   vasopressin
  D   salbutamol
  E   indomethacin

(Answers overleaf)

1.68 A **False** Dominant genes are generally inherited from one
      B **True**   parent, although sporadic mutations are common
      C **False** and the gene may not appear in preceding
      D **False** generations. Siblings have a 1 in 2 chance of being
      E **True**   affected. If a child does not have the gene (i.e. is
                    unaffected) it cannot pass it on. Penetrance, or
                    expression of the genotype in the phenotype is
                    often variable.

1.69 A **False** Adrenogenital syndrome is inherited via an
      B **True**   autosomal gene and achondroplasia is via an
      C **False** autosomal dominant. Turner's syndrome is due to
      D **True**   an absence of one sex chromosome (45X0).
      E **False**

1.70 A **False** Down syndrome, trisomy 21, is usually caused by
      B **False** non-disjunction during meiosis, leaving one germ
      C **True**   cell with two chromosome 21s and another with
      D **True**   none. Fertilisation with a normal germ cell leads to
      E **False** three chromosome 21s (trisomy). Triploidy is the
                    presence of 69 chromosomes. In most cases,
                    therefore, the maternal and paternal karyotypes are
                    normal, but in a few cases (about 5%) one or other
                    partner has a balanced translocation involving
                    chromosome 21 which leads to an increase in the
                    genetic material in the affected child without
                    altering the chromosome number.

1.71 A **False** Haemophilia is an X-linked disease inherited from
      B **True**   the mother, not the father who will be normal.
      C **True**   Similarly, an individual's sons will not be affected,
      D **True**   but his daughters will all inherit his X chromosome
      E **False** and be carriers. His sisters will have inherited one
                    of his mother's X chromosomes, and hence have a
                    50% chance of being affected.

1.72 A **True**   Tocolytics relax the myometrium. Magnesium
      B **True**   sulphate and nifedipine interfere directly with
      C **False** calcium metabolism and transport. Salbutamol, a β_2
      D **True**   adrenoceptor stimulator does so indirectly.
      E **True**   Indomethacin is a prostaglandin synthetase
                    inhibitor and reduces local production of oxytocic
                    prostaglandins. Vasopressin is structurally similar to
                    oxytocin and causes uterine contraction.

1.73 Ergometrine, when given at delivery
A   causes transient hypertension
B   is antiemetic
C   intramuscularly, works within one minute
D   causes rhythmic uterine contractions
E   reduces postpartum blood loss

1.74 Cyproterone acetate
A   binds to androgen receptors
B   is safe to use in early pregnancy
C   is used to treat hirsutism
D   is a contraceptive
E   causes acne

1.75 The following drugs reduce the efficacy of combined oral contraceptives
A   digoxin
B   rifampicin
C   phenytoin
D   ampicillin
E   diazepam

1.76 *Neisseria gonorrhoeae*
A   is a diplococcus
B   is usually found extracellularly
C   is a commensal in the nasopharynx
D   may be detected by fluorescent-staining
E   is a commensal in the rectum

1.77 *Candida albicans*
A   is an anaerobe
B   is a commensal in the bowel
C   has flagellae
D   is Gram-positive
E   colonies appear as sulphur granules

1.78 The neonatal mortality rate
A   only includes deaths in the first week of life
B   includes all deaths in the first four weeks of life
C   does not include infants born at less than 24 weeks gestation
D   is expressed as deaths per 1000 live births
E   is deaths in the first year of life per 1000 live births

(Answers overleaf)

1.73 A **True**   Ergometrine causes vasoconstriction and
     B **False**   hypertension as well as causing tonic uterine
     C **False**   contraction and increasing circulating blood volume
     D **False**   by moving blood from the uterus into the
     E **True**   circulation. The contraction of the myometrium
                   constricts placental bed vessels and reduces blood
                   loss. Gut smooth muscle also contracts and
                   patients usually vomit. Given I.M. it takes
                   approximately seven minutes to work.

1.74 A **True**   Cyproterone acetate binds to androgen receptors
     B **False**   and acts as a competitive inhibitor. It is used to
     C **True**   treat hirsutism and is likely to make acne better.
     D **False**   Patients need to be warned that it is not an effective
     E **False**   contraceptive and is teratogenic so they must use
                   an effective contraceptive when taking the drug.

1.75 A **False**   Rifampicin increases the rate of metabolism of
     B **True**   combined oral contraceptives, as does phenytoin.
     C **True**   The contraceptive effect of oral preparations is
     D **True**   reduced when taking broad spectrum antibiotics
     E **False**   such as ampicillin or tetracycline, although the risk
                   of pregnancy is small.

1.76 A **True**   *Neisseria gonorrhoeae* is an intracellular
     B **False**   diplococcus that is not a commensal anywhere. It
     C **False**   can be detected by fluorescent staining.
     D **True**
     E **False**

1.77 A **False**   *Candida albicans*, responsible for thrush, is a
     B **True**   Gram-positive aerobic organism that is not
     C **False**   flagellate. It is a common commensal in the bowel.
     D **True**   Sulphur granules are characteristic of Actinomyces.
     E **False**

1.78 A **False**   The neonatal mortality rate includes all deaths in
     B **True**   the first four weeks after delivery, regardless of the
     C **False**   gestation at delivery. It is expressed as a rate per
     D **True**   1000 live births.
     E **False**

1.79 The stillbirth rate

A   does not include fetuses dying in utero before 24 weeks gestation

B   includes any infant born dead after 24 weeks gestation

C   is expressed as deaths per 1000 pregnancies

D   includes all cases of abortion

E   includes neonates born alive weighing less than 500 g

1.80 The perinatal mortality rate

A   is the number of stillbirths and neonatal deaths per 1000 live births

B   is the number of stillbirths and deaths in the first week of life per 1000 total births

C   excludes major congenital abnormalities

D   includes all abortions after 20 weeks gestation

E   does not include first week deaths of infants weighing less than 500 g

(Answers overleaf)

1.79 A   **False**   Stillbirths include all babies born dead after
      B   **True**   24 weeks gestation, whenever the death occurred.
      C   **False**   Abortions occurring before 24 weeks are not
      D   **False**   included and neither are babies showing signs of
      E   **False**   life at birth, whatever their weight. It is expressed
                      as a rate per 1000 total births.

1.80 A   **False**   The perinatal mortality rate includes all stillbirths,
      B   **True**   babies born dead after 24 weeks, and all first week
      C   **False**   deaths. Any baby showing signs of life at birth who
      D   **False**   dies within seven days is included. It is expressed
      E   **False**   as a number per 1000 total births (live and dead).

2. Gynaecology

PELVIC PAIN AND INFECTION

2.1 Vaginal trichomonal infection
- A is caused by a flagellated protozoan
- B causes a frothy vaginal discharge
- C is usually sexually transmitted
- D may cause abnormal cervical cytology
- E is treated with metronidazole

2.2 The following investigations may be useful in diagnosing infection with *Trichomonas vaginalis*
- A culture of vaginal secretions
- B microscopic examination of diluted vaginal secretions
- C an eosinophil count in the patient's blood
- D cervical cytology
- E examination of urinary sediment

2.3 Candidiasis of the vulva and vagina occur more frequently in patients who are
- A given long term antibiotic therapy
- B diabetic
- C thyrotoxic
- D taking the oral contraceptive pill
- E pregnant

2.4 Vaginal candidiasis
- A may be diagnosed by cervical cytology
- B is characteristically associated with a frothy green discharge
- C may be sexually transmitted
- D is usually treated with oral nystatin
- E is premalignant

2.5 The natural defences of the vagina to infection include
- A the vaginal pH
- B the presence of Döderlein's bacilli
- C the physical apposition of the pudendal cleft and the vaginal walls
- D the bacteriostatic secretions of vaginal glands
- E the vaginal stratified squamous epithelium

(Answers overleaf)

PELVIC PAIN AND INFECTION

2.1   A   **True**   *Trichomonas vaginalis* is a protozoan which is
      B   **True**   frequently sexually transmitted. Infection is
      C   **True**   localised to the vagina and cervix and does not
      D   **True**   extend to cause salpingitis. An inflammatory
      E   **True**   cervical smear may appear similar to that of mild
                     dysplasia. This must be repeated following
                     treatment. Treatment is with metronidazole 400 mg
                     three times a day for one week. It is important to
                     treat both partners.

2.2   A   **True**   Trichomoniasis can be diagnosed by seeing the
      B   **True**   protozoan on microscopy of diluted vaginal
      C   **False**   secretions or on a cervical smear and after culture
      D   **True**   and Gram staining of the secretions or urinary
      E   **True**   sediment. Eosinophilia does not occur.

2.3   A   **True**   Candidiasis is more frequent in patients with high
      B   **True**   oestrogen levels, e.g. pregnancy or on the oral
      C   **False**   contraceptive pill. It is also more frequent in those
      D   **True**   who have glycosuria or who have the vaginal
      E   **True**   bacterial flora altered by antibiotics.

2.4   A   **True**   Vaginal candidiasis is characterised by a thick,
      B   **False**   white discharge. It is not a venereal disease but
      C   **True**   may be sexually transmitted and is not
      D   **False**   premalignant. The organisms may be seen on
      E   **False**   cervical smears. Treatment is either with imidazole
                      preparations such as clotrimazole which can be
                      given as a single pessary or nystatin creams or
                      pessaries. Nystatin is not absorbed when taken by
                      mouth.

2.5   A   **True**   The acid vaginal pH and relatively impermeable
      B   **True**   squamous epithelium together with the normal
      C   **True**   flora of the vagina all contribute to keeping
      D   **False**   pathogens at bay. There are no vaginal glands.
      E   **True**   Menstruation increases vaginal pH transiently.

2.6 Vaginal discharge causing pruritus vulvae is commonly due to
A Trichomonas vaginalis
B Escherichia coli
C Candida albicans
D Gardnerella vaginalis
E Listeria monocytogenes

2.7 Gardnerella vaginalis vaginitis
A is usually asymptomatic
B may present with a foul smelling discharge
C may progress to acute pelvic inflammatory disease
D should always be treated
E can be diagnosed by 'clue cells' on Gram staining of vaginal discharge

2.8 Gonorrhoea
A is caused by a Gram-negative intracellular diplococcus
B is frequently associated with Trichomonas vaginalis
C is transferred from person to person by fomites
D is often asymptomatic in women
E frequently leads to infertility

2.9 An infected Bartholin's cyst
A is usually bilateral
B is often asymptomatic
C may be caused by an underlying carcinoma
D is most commonly caused by Neisseria gonorrhoeae
E is best treated conservatively with antibiotics

2.10 Condylomata accuminata
A are caused by the papilloma virus
B can be transmitted at sexual intercourse
C often regress during pregnancy
D can be treated with topical idoxuridine
E frequently cause pruritis and discharge

2.11 Vulvovaginitis in a child
A is usually caused by Candida albicans
B occurs because of a lack of the alkaline secretions in the vagina
C may be gonococcal
D is frequently caused by a foreign body in the vagina
E may be caused by thread worms

(Answers overleaf)

2.6   A   **True**   Pruritic discharges can be due to *Trichomonas*
     B   **False**   *vaginalis* or *Candida albicans*. The other organisms
     C   **True**   cause vulval soreness but not pruritus.
     D   **False**
     E   **False**

2.7   A   **True**   *Gardnerella vaginalis* (previously known as
     B   **True**   haemophylis vaginalis) infection is reported
     C   **False**   frequently in asymptomatic patients who have had
     D   **False**   cervical smears taken. Clue cells are vaginal
     E   **True**   epithelial cells covered with small Gram-negative
bacteria and diagnose the condition. The infection
may become symptomatic when there is usually a
foul smelling discharge, and occasional pruritus or
a burning sensation. In the absence of
symptomatology it is not necessary to treat the
infection.

2.8   A   **True**   The Gram-negative intracellular diplococcus
     B   **True**   *Neisseria gonorrhoeae* is almost invariably
     C   **False**   transmitted by direct contact, particularly sexual
     D   **True**   contact and is frequently associated with other
     E   **True**   common sexually transmitted diseases such as
trichomoniasis. It is often asymptomatic, but if
salpingitis is caused, frequently leads to tubal
damage and infertility.

2.9   A   **False**   A Bartholin's abscess is unilateral, very painful and
     B   **False**   best treated surgically by incision, drainage and
     C   **True**   marsupialisation. Very infrequently there may be an
     D   **False**   underlying carcinoma. Most cases are due to
     E   **False**   infection with coliform bacteria.

2.10 A   **True**   Condylomata accuminata are genital warts caused
     B   **True**   by the papilloma virus. They are sexually
     C   **False**   transmitted, and can be associated with secondary
     D   **False**   infection. They usually grow larger in pregnancy
     E   **True**   but tend to regress after delivery. They can be
treated by topical podophyllin (out of pregnancy) or
if more severe by electrocautery or laser ablation
under an anaesthetic.

2.11 A   **False**   Vulvovaginitis is the commonest gynaecological
     B   **False**   disorder in children. It occurs mainly because of the
     C   **True**   lack of protective acidity in the vagina. The infection
     D   **False**   is usually with a mixed flora. Monilial infection and
     E   **True**   foreign bodies are found relatively rarely. Thread
worms sometimes cause vulvovaginitis as does
gonorrhoea although this is becoming less common.

2.12 Chronic cervicitis
- A is often associated with the presence of Nabothian follicles on the cervix
- B may cause subfertility
- C is usually caused by an anaerobic infection
- D should be treated if asymptomatic
- E can usually be treated by cryocautery as an out-patient

2.13 Acute cervicitis
- A is uncommon
- B usually causes deep dyspareunia
- C is often gonococcal
- D is treated by electrocautery
- E may be herpetic in origin

2.14 Genital tract tuberculosis
- A leads to infertility
- B is often asymptomatic
- C is usually an ascending infection from the vagina
- D always involves the cervix
- E may be diagnosed by histological examination of the endometrium

2.15 Acute pelvic inflammatory disease
- A should be treated with ampicillin and flagyl
- B is frequently due to infection with *Chlamydia trachomatis*
- C is usually diagnosed laparoscopically
- D leads to subsequent infertility in 40% of cases
- E may give rise to signs of peritonism

2.16 Pyometra may be a complication of
- A carcinoma of the endometrium
- B carcinoma of the cervix
- C carcinoma of the vulva
- D radiotherapy
- E acute endometritis

2.17 Acute pelvic inflammatory disease
- A is common in pregnancy
- B is most commonly caused by *Chlamydia trachomatis*
- C is associated with Fitz–Hugh Curtis syndrome
- D is usually bilateral
- E is most common in women between 30 and 35 years of age

(Answers overleaf)

2.12 A **True**   Chronic cervicitis is an extremely common
     B **True**   condition and is often asymptomatic. In more
     C **False** severe forms there is profuse vaginal discharge,
     D **False** chronic sacral backache,. dyspareunia and
     E **True**   occasionally postcoital bleeding. Bacterial culture of
                  the discharge is usually sterile. Subfertility may be
                  caused by a cervical mucus hostility. Chronic
                  cervicitis responds to treatment with cryocautery
                  but this is only necessary if the patient has
                  symptoms.

2.13 A **True**   When acute inflammation of the cervix does occur
     B **False** it is usually gonococcal or herpetic and is often
     C **True**   asymptomatic. Treatment is directed at the cause.
     D **False**
     E **True**

2.14 A **True**   Genital tract tuberculosis is not very common. It is
     B **True**   a descending infection, which always involves the
     C **False** fallopian tubes, sometimes involves the
     D **False** endometrium and rarely involves the cervix. It is
     E **True**   often asymptomatic but often causes infertility. It
                  can be diagnosed by histological examination of
                  the endometrium.

2.15 A **False** Pelvic inflammatory disease is inflammation of the
     B **True**   upper genital tract. Treatment should be with
     C **False** erythromycin or tetracycline and not ampicillin as a
     D **False** broad spectrum antibiotic is required which also
     E **True**   acts against chlamydia. Flagyl is necessary to treat
                  anaerobic infection. Generally the diagnosis is
                  made on clinical grounds but the diagnosis should
                  be confirmed by laparoscopy if the pain does not
                  settle after 24 hours of antibiotics. An acute episode
                  of pelvic infection leads to subsequent infertility in
                  less than 10% of cases.

2.16 A **True**   Development of pyometra depends upon the
     B **True**   development of a cervical stenosis either by
     C **False** carcinoma, or following radiotherapy. Acute
     D **True**   endometritis leads to vaginal discharge.
     E **False**

2.17 A **False** Acute pelvic inflammatory disease is most common
     B **True**   under the age of 25. It is usually bilateral.
     C **True**   *Chlamydia trachomatis* causes more than 50% of
     D **True**   cases of pelvic inflammatory disease and it can be
     E **False** associated with peri-hepatitis which is known as the
                  Fitz–Hugh Curtis syndrome. Due to the mechanical
                  barrier in pregnancy it is extremely rare.

2.18 **Chronic pelvic inflammatory disease**
A is clinically difficult to differentiate from endometriosis
B may cause oligomenorrhoea
C responds well to long term antibiotic therapy
D is best treated by total abdominal hysterectomy and bilateral salpingo-oophorectomy if definitive surgery is required
E commonly causes secondary dysmenorrhoea

2.19 **Endometriosis can be treated with**
A excision of large chocolate cysts
B GNRH analogues
C stilboestrol
D norethisterone for 21 days in each cycle
E hysterectomy and bilateral salpingo-oophorectomy in severe cases

2.20 **Changes that occur in the vagina at puberty include**
A colonisation by Döderlein's bacilli
B an increase in the pH
C glycogenation of the epithelium
D the appearance of glands in the epithelium
E exfoliation of superficial cells with pyknotic nuclei

2.21 **If 800 mg per day of danazol is used for the treatment of endometriosis**
A breakthrough bleeding is commonly a problem
B the treatment can be continued for longer than nine months
C nearly all women will be amenorrhoeic
D there is no need to use additional contraception
E relief of symptoms is common

2.22 **Mild endometriosis**
A is commonly associated with subfertility
B can be treated with provera
C is often asymptomatic
D is best diagnosed by laparoscopy
E should be treated in subfertile couples

(Answers overleaf)

2.18 A **True**   Chronic pelvic inflammatory disease classically
     B **False**   causes menorrhagia with short cycles, secondary
     C **False**   dysmenorrhoea, dyspareunia, chronic pelvic pain
     D **True**   and infertility. Its main differential diagnosis is
     E **True**   endometriosis. It does not show a good response to
                   long term antibiotic treatment but exacerbation
                   should be treated with antibiotics. It often comes to
                   surgical treatment and pelvic clearance, including
                   removal of the ovaries, may be necessary to afford
                   relief of symptoms.

2.19 A **True**   Endometriosis can be treated medically with
     B **True**   progestogens (provera, danazol), continuous oral
     C **False**   contraceptive pill or GNRH analogues. Treatment
     D **False**   should be continued for 3–9 months. In more severe
     E **True**   cases the patient can be treated surgically by ablation
                   of small areas with laser or diathermy, excision of
                   cysts or total abdominal hysterectomy and bilateral
                   salpingo-oophorectomy.

2.20 A **True**   At puberty the vagina comes under the influence of
     B **False**   oestrogens, the pH falls, lacto-bacilli invade and the
     C **True**   epithelium becomes glycogenated and thicker with
     D **False**   exfoliation of superficial cells. There are no glands
     E **True**   in the vagina.

2.21 A **False**   On 800 mg per day of danazol, most women will
     B **False**   become amenorrhoeic and will not get breakthrough
     C **True**   bleeding. Relief of symptoms is common and usually
     D **False**   continues for up to six months after discontinuation
     E **True**   of therapy. Recurrence rates after medical treatment
                   are high. Some women can still ovulate on danazol
                   and so the use of a barrier method of contraception is
                   important. There is a possibility of virilisation of a
                   female fetus if a pregnancy occurs. The drug is not
                   licensed to be used for longer than nine months in
                   view of reported cases of abnormal liver function
                   tests and cholestatic jaundice.

2.22 A **True**   Endometriosis is commonest in voluntarily and
     B **True**   involuntarily infertile women in their early 30s.
     C **True**   10–20% of women with subfertility at laparoscopy will
     D **True**   have mild endometriosis. It is often asymptomatic,
     E **False**   but may present with dysmenorrhoea or dyspareunia.
                   It is best diagnosed by laparoscopy but some recent
                   studies have also shown MRI scan to be effective in
                   early diagnosis. There is no evidence that treating
                   mild endometriosis in subfertile women increases
                   their chance of conception. It can be treated, if
                   symptomatic, with a three month course of provera.

2.23 Endometriosis is
A common outside the pelvis
B treated with high dose progestogens
C frequently pre-malignant
D common in women in social groups 4 and 5
E usually treated by abdominal hysterectomy

2.24 Adenomyosis
A often presents as secondary dysmenorrhoea
B often causes oligomenorrhoea
C is treated with hormone therapy
D is more common in multiparous women
E may undergo sarcomatous change

2.25 Adenomyosis
A is diagnosed at dilatation and curettage
B causes menorrhagia
C causes deep dyspareunia
D is treated by hysterectomy
E is associated with endometriosis in 50% of cases

2.26 In adenomyosis
A the uterus is enlarged
B the uterus is tender
C the uterus contains encapsulated areas of endometrium
D the lesions can be localised or diffusely spread through the uterus
E glandular tissue is found between the uterine muscle fibres

2.27 Superficial dyspareunia may be caused by
A infection with *Trichomonas vaginalis*
B pelvic inflammatory disease
C endometriosis
D adenomyosis
E atrophic vaginitis

2.28 Treatment of severe primary dysmenorrhoea can include
A opiate analgesics
B inhibition of ovulation
C dilatation and curettage
D sympathectomy
E hysterectomy

(Answers overleaf)

2.23 A **False** Endometriotic deposits are only rarely found in the
 B **True** lung and at other extra-pelvic sites. The disease can
 C **False** be suppressed by progestogens or bilateral
 D **False** oophorectomy. Hysterectomy alone is unlikely to
 E **False** help. It is more frequently diagnosed in women of
 social groups 1 and 2. Malignant change may take
 place to endometrioid carcinoma but this is rare.

2.24 A **True** Adenomyosis presents with painful heavy periods
 B **False** in multiparous women in mid to late reproductive
 C **False** life. The diagnosis can only be made with certainty
 D **True** by histological examination of the removed uterus.
 E **False** The cellular elements are epithelial and do not
 undergo sarcomatous change.

2.25 A **False** Adenomyosis causes menorrhagia, secondary
 B **True** dysmenorrhoea and deep dyspareunia and is
 C **True** diagnosed after treatment of these symptoms by
 D **True** hysterectomy. Endometriosis and adenomyosis
 E **False** tend to occur in different groups of patients.

2.26 A **True** In adenomyosis the myometrium is locally or
 B **True** diffusely infiltrated with endometrial tissues,
 C **False** including glandular structures. These react to the
 D **True** cyclical hormonal changes and cause enlargement
 E **True** and tenderness of the uterus.

2.27 A **False** Superficial dyspareunia is pain at the vulva or
 B **False** vagina during sexual intercourse. This can be
 C **False** caused by infection leading to vaginal inflammation
 D **False** or inability of the atrophic epithelium to deal with
 E **True** the trauma of intercourse. Pelvic inflammatory
 disease, endometriosis and adenomyosis cause
 deep dyspareunia.

2.28 A **False** Primary dysmenorrhoea occurs in ovulatory cycles
 B **True** from shortly after the menarche. It can be treated
 C **False** by inhibiting ovulation, by pregnancy or with
 D **False** prostaglandin synthetase inhibitors. The majority of
 E **False** these patients are young and are not candidates for
 surgery, even curettage. In this chronic condition
 opiates would be addictive.

2.29 Secondary dysmenorrhoea
A   may be caused by endometriosis
B   is treated by dilatation and curettage
C   is commonest in women aged between 20 and 25 years
D   is often associated with organic pathology in the pelvis
E   is usually treated with the oral contraceptive pill

2.30 Common causes of chronic pelvic pain include
A   pelvic infection
B   irritable bowel syndrome
C   ovarian cancer
D   uterine fibroids
E   uterine retroversion

HORMONAL AND MENSTRUAL PROBLEMS

2.31 In a woman of 38 years complaining of heavy periods
A   measured blood loss of greater than 80 ml per period is
    likely to lead to anaemia
B   a pathological cause is found at hysterectomy in most
    cases
C   a dilatation and curettage should be performed
D   an out-patient hysteroscopy should be performed
E   she will most frequently have regular ovulatory cycles

2.32 Complications of dilatation and curettage include
A   uterine perforation
B   cervical laceration
C   cervical stenosis
D   Asherman's syndrome
E   endometritis

(Answers overleaf)

2.29 A **True**   Secondary dysmenorrhoea is painful periods
     B **False** occurring after pain free periods. It commonly occurs
     C **False** in women in their thirties and is frequently secondary
     D **True**   to pelvic pathology such as endometriosis or
     E **False** adenomyosis. Curettage is a diagnostic procedure
                and rarely helps. Treatment should be aimed at the
                underlying cause and is often surgical.

2.30 A **True**   Fibroids and ovarian tumours rarely cause pelvic pain
     B **True**   except as a late phenomenon. Uterine retroversion
     C **False** occurs in 15% of women and is almost invariably
     D **False** innocent. Pelvic infection is the commonest
     E **False** gynaecological cause of pelvic pain, although the
                irritable bowel syndrome may be the commonest
                overall.

HORMONAL AND MENSTRUAL PROBLEMS

2.31 A **True**   Although most women who have a measured blood
     B **False** loss of greater than 80 ml per period are likely to
     C **False** become anaemic, only 40% of women who complain
     D **True**   of flooding or passage of clots actually lose more than
     E **True**   80 ml per cycle. A dilatation and curettage is a
                diagnostic procedure and not a therapeutic
                procedure. Therefore unless there are additional
                symptoms like intermenstrual bleeding there is no
                value in performing this procedure before the age of
                40 years. There is, however, recent evidence that an
                out-patient hysteroscopy to detect endometrial
                polyps and submucous fibroids is a much more
                valuable procedure. Most women with menorrhagia
                have regular ovulatory cycle although menorrhagia
                can occur in anovulatory cycles either shortly after the
                menarche or just prior to the menopause.

2.32 A **True**   Complications of curettage include trauma,
     B **True**   perforation or cervical tear which may itself lead to
     C **True**   scarring and stenosis, curetting the basal layer and
     D **True**   causing intrauterine adhesions to form (Asherman's
     E **True**   syndrome, and introducing infection).

2.33 A 40-year-old woman with dysfunctional bleeding may require treatment with
A endometrial ablation
B oral contraceptive preparations
C tranexamic acid
D clomiphene citrate
E mefenamic acid

2.34 A 40-year-old woman with intermenstrual bleeding
A should be given an oral progestogen
B should have a diagnostic curettage
C is probably perimenopausal
D may have cervical cancer
E can be treated with dicynene if her cervical cytology is normal

2.35 Metropathia haemorrhagica
A is seen most frequently at the extremes of reproductive age
B means light, frequent uterine bleeding
C only occurs in ovulatory cycles
D can be treated with progestogens
E is associated with cystic hyperplasia of the endometrium

2.36 The following procedures can be performed laparoscopically
A Pommeroy sterilization
B removal of an ectopic pregnancy
C oophorectomy
D tubal surgery
E ventrosuspension

2.37 Ambiguous genitalia at birth
A may be due to congenital adrenal hyperplasia
B can be caused by maternal ingestion of danazol during pregnancy
C occurs in complete androgen insensitivity
D may occur in true hermaphroditism
E the karyotype is nearly always 46 XX

2.38 Precocious puberty
A is most commonly idiopathic
B if idiopathic, does not lead to any long term problems
C may be caused by an ovarian tumour
D is associated with 47 XXX genotype
E may be caused by a cerebral tumour

(Answers overleaf)

2.33 A **True**   Medical treatment of dysfunctional uterine bleeding
      B **True**   includes non-hormonal drugs (mefenamic acid,
      C **True**   tranexamic acid and ethamsylate) and hormonal
      D **False**   drugs (the oral contraceptive pill, progestogen and
      E **True**   GnRH analogues). Surgical treatment includes
                     hysterectomy and endometrial ablative techniques.

2.34 A **False**   Intermenstrual bleeding is commonly due to uterine
      B **True**   pathology and in a 40-year-old woman should
      C **False**   always lead to diagnostic curettage and
      D **True**   hysteroscopy and cervical cytology to exclude
      E **False**   carcinomas of the endometrium and cervix,
                     endometrial polyps and submucous fibroids.

2.35 A **True**   Anovulatory cycles leading to metropathia
      B **False**   haemorrhagica occur most commonly around the
      C **False**   menarche and the menopause. Heavy infrequent
      D **True**   bleeding ensues, best treated with progestogens to
      E **True**   induce secretory changes in the hyperplastic
                     endometrium.

2.36 A **False**   There have been great strides forwards in 'keyhole
      B **True**   surgery' over the last few years. Small ectopics can
      C **True**   be removed by linear salpingotomy, ovaries and
      D **True**   ovarian cysts can be removed. It is possible to
      E **True**   perform tubal surgery with adhesiolysis and
                     salpingostomies using diathermy or laser. The
                     laparoscope can also be used to assist at a vaginal
                     hysterectomy.

2.37 A **True**   Ambiguous genitalia at birth can be due to either a
      B **True**   masculinised female, an undermasculinised male or
      C **False**   a true hermaphrodite. Congenital adrenal
      D **True**   hyperplasia or maternal ingestion of danazol may
      E **False**   cause virilisation of a female fetus. Complete
                     androgen insensitivity presents with primary
                     amenorrhoea in a phenotypically normal female.
                     Only partial androgen insensitivity will present at
                     birth with ambiguous genitalia. The karyotype can
                     be 46 XY, 46 XX or mosaicism.

2.38 A **True**   Precocious puberty is idiopathic in over 95% of
      B **False**   cases. Precocious puberty from whatever cause can
      C **True**   lead to short stature. Oestrogen secreting ovarian
      D **False**   tumours and central nervous system disease such
      E **True**   as pineal tumours, meningitis or encephalitis may
                     lead to precocious puberty. A 47 XXX genotype
                     may lead to delayed puberty.

2.39 At puberty

A menarche usually occurs between the ages of 11 and 15 years

B thelarche (breast development) is the first externally noticeable sign

C axillary hair precedes pubic hair growth

D the girl has usually reached a weight of 45 kg

E the long bone epiphyses close

2.40 Primary amenorrhoea may be due to

A hypoplasia and failure of fusion of the Mullerian ducts

B congenital adrenal hyperplasia

C granulosa cell tumours of the ovary

D endometrial carcinoma

E Kallmann's syndrome

2.41 Investigations of a child presenting with primary amenorrhoea should include a

A serum LH estimation

B serum FSH estimation

C skull X-ray

D karyotype

E diagnostic curettage

2.42 Hirsutism

A is frequently genetically determined

B may be caused by the polycystic ovarian syndrome

C is made worse by shaving

D will improve over 4–6 weeks with the oral contraceptive pill

E may be treated with spironolactone

2.43 Signs of virilism include

A excessive body hair

B occipital balding

C menorrhagia

D clitoromegaly

E muscle development

2.44 Causes of virilism in females include

A congenital adrenal hyperplasia

B Addison's disease

C panhypopituitarism

D hilus cell tumours of the ovary

E arrhenoblastoma

(Answers overleaf)

2.39 A **True**   At puberty breast development occurs first, then
      B **True**   pubic hair and then the axillary hair growth.
      C **False** Menstruation starts at an average of approximately
      D **True**   13 years and appears to be loosely related to
      E **False** weight. Epiphyses close some years later, causing
                    growth to cease.

2.40 A **True**   Mullerian duct hyperplasia accounts for 12% of
      B **True**   cases of primary amenorrhoea. In congenital
      C **False** adrenal hyperplasia the adrenal androgens
      D **False** suppress normal female puberty. Kallmann's
      E **True**   syndrome is isolated gonadotrophin deficiency.
                    Granulosa cell tumours secrete oestrogens and
                    endometrial cancers cause postmenopausal or
                    intermenstrual bleeding.

2.41 A **False** The most important investigation is the serum FSH
      B **True**   which divides the causes of primary amenorrhoea
      C **True**   into the major categories. A karyotype should always
      D **True**   be performed but is most valuable in
      E **False** hypergonadotrophic amenorrhoea. In
                    hypogonadotrophic amenorrhoea, lesions can
                    sometimes be seen on skull X-ray, such as pituitary
                    tumours. Examination under anaesthesia but not
                    curettage may be of value.

2.42 A **True**   Hirsutism, if idiopathic, is commonly genetically or
      B **True**   racially determined. It may be caused by the
      C **False** polycystic ovarian syndrome. It may be treated
      D **False** topically by shaving, waxing, bleaching or the use of
      E **True**   depilatory creams. Shaving does not increase hair
                    growth but it does tend to make hairs coarser.
                    Treatment with hormonal medication, like the oral
                    contraceptive pill, will usually take about six months
                    to have an effect. Spironolactone can be effectively
                    used to treat hirsutism but it is not licensed for this
                    use in the United Kingdom.

2.43 A **True**   Virilism is characterised by excessive body and
      B **False** facial hair, oligomenorrhoea, temporal balding,
      C **False** muscle development, clitoromegaly and deepening
      D **True**   of the voice.
      E **True**

2.44 A **True**   Virilism is due to excess androgens and can be
      B **False** caused by ovarian or adrenal pathology including
      C **False** congenital adrenal hyperplasia, Cushing's
      D **True**   syndrome, adrenal tumours and androgen secreting
      E **True**   ovarian tumours.

2.45 A negative progestogen challenge test
A suggests low endogenous oestrogen levels
B suggests ovulation induction with clomiphene citrate should be effective
C would usually occur in polycystic ovarian syndrome
D may occur in Asherman's syndrome
E may occur in ovarian failure

2.46 Hyperprolactinaemia
A is diagnosed if the serum prolactin concentration is greater than 600 mIu/l
B is usually treated surgically
C can be caused by tricyclic antidepressants
D is usually caused by a pituitary macroadenoma
E should be investigated by CT scan

2.47 Polycystic ovarian syndrome
A is always diagnosed by ultrasound scan
B is associated with an increased risk of endometrial cancer
C is associated with obesity
D if associated with amenorrhoea should always be treated
E if associated with hirsutism can be treated by the oral contraceptive pill

2.48 The following serum hormone concentrations are usually increased in polycystic ovarian syndrome
A LH
B FSH
C oestradiol
D prolactin
E SHBG

(Answers overleaf)

2.45 A **True** A progestogen challenge test is usually performed
B **False** by giving provera 10 mg a day for five days in an
C **False** amenorrhoeic woman. A negative result suggests
D **True** low endogenous oestrogen levels. Ovulation
E **True** induction would therefore usually require the use of
gonadotrophins and anti-oestrogens are usually not
effective. Women with polycystic ovarian syndrome
commonly have normal oestrogen level and
therefore have a positive test result.

2.46 A **False** Serum prolactin concentration needs to be over
B **False** 1000 mIu/l before a diagnosis of hyperprolactinaemia
C **True** can be made. The usual cause is a pituitary
D **False** microadenoma and it is only rarely due to a pituitary
E **True** macroadenoma. All patients should be investigated
by CT scan to see the size of the tumour, if one is
present, and to exclude any pituitary stalk
compression from extrinsic lesions. Once extrinsic
compression of the pituitary stalk has been excluded
most patients respond to medical treatment with
bromocriptine.

2.47 A **False** Some women with polycystic ovarian syndrome
B **True** have classic symptoms and signs of polycystic
C **True** ovarian syndrome with biochemical evidence of the
D **True** condition but a normal ultrasound scan. Because of
E **True** the high unopposed oestrogens in this condition
there is an increased risk of endometrial cancer,
breast cancer and cardiovascular disease. For these
reasons oestrogens should be opposed with
progestogens. If associated with hirsutism giving
oestrogens as well may raise the SHBG level and
so suppress the free androgen concentration in the
blood which may lead to a decrease in hair growth.

2.48 A **True** The classic endocrine changes in polycystic ovarian
B **False** syndrome are of a high early follicular LH level with
C **False** a normal or low FSH level. This gives rise to the
D **False** high LH to FSH ratio. Oestradiol levels are often
E **False** normal or can be low. Total oestrogen levels are
often high due to the high oestrone levels that are
present. Prolactin is usually normal although it can
occasionally be raised. Sex hormone binding
globulin levels are usually suppressed by the high
androgen concentrations. This means that even if
androgen concentrations are normal free androgen
levels are often very high.

2.49 Turner's syndrome is associated with

   A   normal breast development
   B   an absent uterus
   C   primary amenorrhoea
   D   hirsutism
   E   streak ovaries

2.50 Causes of delayed puberty include

   A   myxoedema
   B   an imperforate hymen
   C   congenital absence of the uterus
   D   Turner's syndrome
   E   Klinefelter's syndrome

2.51 Premature menopause is associated with

   A   a lowered FSH concentration
   B   chromosomal abnormality
   C   secondary amenorrhoea
   D   uterine leiomyomata
   E   chemotherapy

2.52 Investigation of secondary amenorrhoea should include

   A   serum testosterone estimation
   B   a karyotype
   C   a pelvic ultrasound scan
   D   serum prolactin concentration
   E   FSH estimation

2.53 Secondary amenorrhoea may be due to

   A   polycystic ovarian syndrome
   B   endometriosis
   C   resistant ovarian syndrome
   D   anorexia nervosa
   E   Asherman's syndrome

(Answers overleaf)

2.49 A **False** In Turner's syndrome (XO) there is usually ovarian
B **False** failure with streak ovaries and primary amenorrhoea.
C **True** Mullerian duct structures are, however, present. The
D **False** lack of oestrogen causes failure of breast
E **True** development but there are no excess androgens so
virilism does not occur. If the karyotype is a
45XO/46XX mosaic, some women have periods and
then develop a premature menopause.

2.50 A **False** Delayed puberty in females means failure of
B **False** development of secondary sexual characteristics as
C **False** well as amenorrhoea. Consequently anatomical
D **True** problems will not delay puberty. Turner's syndrome
E **True** prevents puberty occurring. Juvenile myxoedema
may lead to precocious puberty (although rarely
Hashimoto's disease in children may cause delay). In
males, Klinefelter's syndrome may lead to delayed
puberty depending on the androgen concentrations
achieved.

2.51 A **False** Premature menopause is usually defined as
B **True** menopause before the age of 35 years of age. Women
C **True** develop secondary amenorrhoea associated with a
D **False** high serum FSH concentration. It is associated with
E **True** chemotherapy, radiotherapy, chromosomal
abnormalities (Turner's mosaics), the development of
ovarian antibodies and infections (e.g. mumps).

2.52 A **True** A serum testosterone level of less than 5 nmol/l will
B **False** exclude a virilising tumour of the ovary or adrenal. An
C **True** FSH if it is high will suggest premature menopause or
D **True** resistant ovary syndrome. An ultrasound scan is
E **True** helpful in diagnosing polycystic ovarian syndrome
and excluding tumours of the ovary. A karyotype is
unnecessary in the investigation of secondary
amenorrhoea but important in primary amenorrhoea.

2.53 A **True** Secondary amenorrhoea may be caused by
B **False** hypothalamic factors like the weight change of
C **True** anorexia nervosa. Ovarian causes include polycystic
D **True** ovarian syndrome and resistant ovary syndrome.
E **True** Endometriosis does not cause amenorrhoea.
Asherman's syndrome where the uterine cavity is
obliterated following a curettage of the uterus can
also lead to secondary amenorrhoea.

2.54 The premenstrual syndrome includes

A a feeling of abdominal distension
B pelvic pain immediately before menstruation
C premenstrual irritability and depression
D failure to ovulate
E tender breasts

2.55 The premenstrual syndrome

A is associated with premenstrual weight gain
B is best treated with diuretics
C is frequently associated with changes in girth
D is associated with alterations in perceived body image
E may be treated by dydrogesterone

2.56 In a woman's blood after the menopause

A FSH levels rise
B most of the circulating oestrogen is in the form of oestrone
C oestradiol levels fall
D androstenedione levels increase
E the quantity of oestrogens present is increased by obesity

2.57 Hormone replacement therapy

A can reverse osteoporosis
B is contraindicated in hypertension
C prevents menopausal flushes
D must be given orally
E usually causes amenorrhoea

2.58 When treating menopausal symptoms

A norethisterone acetate is effective
B ethinyl oestradiol may cause endometrial carcinoma
C therapy is rarely needed for more than four months
D counselling and reassurance may be as effective as any drug therapy
E withdrawal bleeding following a combined oestrogen and progesterone preparation is not an indication for curettage

2.59 Menorrhagia is associated with

A adenomyosis
B endometriosis
C chronic pelvic infection
D resistant ovary syndrome
E hypothyroidism

(Answers overleaf)

2.54 A **True**   True premenstrual syndrome occurs in ovulatory
     B **False**   cycles and is frequently characterised with
     C **True**   distension, irritability and breast tenderness.
     D **False**   Although pelvic pain may be present as well,
     E **True**   premenstrual syndrome should not be confused
            with dysmenorrhoea.

2.55 A **False**   In trials performed on patients with premenstrual
     B **False**   syndrome there is no evidence for widespread
     C **False**   weight gain, fluid retention or changes in girth
     D **True**   premenstrually despite anecdotal evidence. A
     E **True**   change is noted, however, in perception of girth. As
            there is no evidence of fluid retention diuretics are
            an illogical treatment. Dydrogesterone frequently
            works but then so do many placebos. The aetiology
            of this condition remains obscure.

2.56 A **True**   After the menopause ovarian oestradiol production
     B **True**   falls. Androstenedione is produced by the adrenal,
     C **True**   but the plasma concentration is only half that of the
     D **False**   woman of reproductive age. Androstenedione is
     E **True**   aromatised to oestrone, particularly in adipose
            tissue. As oestrogen levels fall FSH increases.

2.57 A **False**   Hormone replacement therapy can be given orally,
     B **False**   transdermally or as subcutaneous implants. It will
     C **True**   prevent menopausal symptoms including hot
     D **False**   flushes. Most women using combined hormone
     E **False**   replacement therapy will continue to have regular
            withdrawal bleeds. It can prevent osteoporosis but
            will not reverse any changes that have already
            occurred. It can be used in controlled hypertension.

2.58 A **False**   Oestrogens and sympathy are the treatment of
     B **True**   choice for menopausal symptoms. Because of the
     C **False**   oestrogen effect on the endometrium, causing
     D **True**   hyperplasia and potentially malignancy, a combined
     E **True**   preparation is best. Therapy should continue for
            6–12 months in the first instance. Any bleeding
            apart from regular monthly withdrawal bleeds is an
            indication for curettage.

2.59 A **True**   Fibroids, adenomyosis, endometriosis, chronic
     B **True**   pelvic infection and hypothyroidism are all
     C **True**   associated with menorrhagia. Resistant ovary
     D **False**   syndrome is a cause of secondary amenorrhoea.
     E **True**

2.60 Concerning the climacteric

A   it is symptomatic in greater than 50% of women
B   it is the time at which menstruation ceases
C   oestrogen is the only effective drug treatment available
D   it is best managed under consultant care
E   it is commonly associated with sexual dysfunction

PROLAPSE AND URINARY PROBLEMS

2.61 Prolapse is associated with

A   obesity
B   chronic bronchitis
C   excessive coitus
D   inguinal hernia
E   carcinoma of the cervix

2.62 Second degree uterine prolapse

A   can be diagnosed when the cervix protrudes through the vulval orifice
B   is also known as complete procidentia
C   may present with menorrhagia
D   causes lumbar backache
E   causes sacral backache

2.63 Structures which prevent prolapse of the uterus and vagina include the

A   round ligaments
B   levator ani muscle
C   uterosacral ligaments
D   cardinal ligaments
E   broad ligaments

2.64 Factors predisposing to the development of uterovaginal prolapse include

A   congenital weakness of the supporting ligaments
B   postmenopausal atrophy
C   endometrial polyps
D   ovarian tumours
E   injury during childbirth

(Answers overleaf)

2.60 A **True**   The climacteric is the transitional period during
     B **False** which a woman's reproductive capacity ceases.
     C **False** Three-quarters of women will have symptoms and
     D **False** one-third of those may have severe symptoms. It is
     E **True**   easily managed in general practice in the majority
                   of cases. The commonest symptoms are
                   vasomotor, e.g. hot flushes, emotional changes
                   including loss of libido and often urinary
                   symptoms. Clonidine may reduce vasomotor
                   symptoms and is useful if oestrogens are
                   contraindicated.

PROLAPSE AND URINARY PROBLEMS

2.61 A **True**   Prolapse is caused by weakness of the supports of
     B **True**   the uterus. The cervical ligaments are either
     C **False** congenitally weak, or have been stretched at
     D **False** childbirth. Causes of raised intra-abdominal
     E **False** pressure, including obesity, chronic bronchitis and
                   chronic constipation make matters worse.

2.62 A **True**   Second degree uterine prolapse is diagnosed when
     B **False** the cervix protrudes through the vulva. If all of the
     C **False** uterus comes out this is third degree prolapse, also
     D **False** known as complete procidentia. Prolapse presents
     E **True**   with sacral backache, lumbar backache is
                   musculoskeletal, and does not cause alterations in
                   menstruation.

2.63 A **False** The major supports are the uterosacral and
     B **True**   transverse cervical (cardinal) ligaments and
     C **True**   tightening of these is the most important step in
     D **True**   surgery for uterine prolapse.
     E **False**

2.64 A **True**   Anything that weakens the cervical ligaments will
     B **True**   predispose to uterine prolapse. Congenital
     C **False** weakness, injury and atrophy after the menopause
     D **False** are the main causes. Ovarian tumours increase the
     E **True**   pressure in the abdomen but as they get larger
                   they rise out of the pelvis and pull the uterus up.

2.65 Backache associated with uterine prolapse

A is usually sacral
B occurs mainly at night in bed
C is caused by traction on the uterosacral ligaments
D is accompanied by tenderness in the lumbar region
E is often due to coincidental musculoskeletal problems

2.66 Long term complications of uterovaginal prolapse may include

A uraemia
B bladder instability
C vaginal ulceration
D endometrial carcinoma
E vulval atrophy

2.67 A patient with uterovaginal prolapse

A is usually nulliparous
B is usually premenopausal
C often complains of dyspareunia
D may present with a purulent bloody discharge
E may complain of stress incontinence

2.68 Treatment with a ring pessary for vaginal prolapse is generally indicated in patients

A more than 75 years old
B wishing to become pregnant
C who refuse operation
D who have pre-existing vaginal ulceration
E in the puerperium

2.69 The 'Manchester' repair includes

A vaginal hysterectomy
B amputation of the cervix
C anterior colporrhaphy
D faradic stimulation
E posterior colpoperineorrhaphy

2.70 An enterocele

A usually contains rectum
B is lined by peritoneum
C frequently contains small bowel
D may be a long-term complication of vaginal hysterectomy
E is usually diagnosed by barium enema

(Answers overleaf)

2.65 A **True**   Many women in the age group that has
      B **False**   uterovaginal prolapse will have coincidental
      C **True**   musculoskeletal problems, particularly lumbar
      D **False**   backache. Prolapse and traction on the ligaments
      E **True**   causes sacral backache which is completely relieved
                     by lying down.

2.66 A **True**   Long term prolapse may lead to ureteric kinking,
      B **True**   hydronephrosis and uraemia. Urethral obstruction
      C **True**   leads to incomplete bladder emptying, urinary
      D **False**   stasis, infection and bladder instability. Ulceration
      E **False**   may occur at the site of the most dependent part of
                     the prolapse. This is followed by discharge and
                     vulval soreness, not atrophy. Very occasionally
                     cervical cancer complicates prolapse.

2.67 A **False**   Uterovaginal prolapse is most common in
      B **False**   multiparous postmenopausal women. If symptoms
      C **False**   are present the complaints are usually of
      D **True**   'something coming down' backache and stress
      E **True**   incontinence or, a bloody discharge if ulceration
                     has occurred. Dyspareunia is uncommon.

2.68 A **False**   The treatment of choice for all patients with
      B **False**   prolapse is surgery unless they are exceptionally
      C **True**   unfit, refuse an operation or it is expected that the
      D **False**   ligaments will tighten spontaneously, as in the
      E **True**   puerperium.

2.69 A **False**   A Manchester operation includes anterior
      B **True**   colporrhaphy, amputation of the cervix and
      C **True**   posterior colpoperineorrhaphy. The most important
      D **False**   step is shortening of the cervical ligaments. Faradic
      E **True**   stimulation is electrical stimulation of the muscles
                     of the pelvic floor.

2.70 A **False**   An enterocele is a prolapse of the pouch of
      B **True**   Douglas, containing peritoneum and sometimes
      C **True**   small bowel. It is the commonest recurrent prolapse
      D **True**   after vaginal hysterectomy. A prolapse containing
      E **False**   rectum is a rectocele. The diagnosis is clinical,
                     rectal examination separates an enterocele from a
                     rectocele.

2.71 A cystocele
A is always associated with stress incontinence
B contains bladder
C may present as urinary retention
D is often asymptomatic
E is best treated with a ring pessary

2.72 Asymptomatic bacteriuria
A is associated with a colony count of 100 000 per ml of urine
B is usually due to *Escherichia coli*
C is often due to anaerobic organisms
D is always accompanied by pyuria
E occurs in 15% of all women of reproductive age

2.73 Stress incontinence can be caused by
A multiple sclerosis
B alteration of the urethrovesical angle
C a rectocele
D myasthenia gravis
E a cystourethrocele

2.74 Stress incontinence
A is associated with obliteration of the posterior urethrovesical angle
B means having to pass urine frequently
C occurs in all cases of severe uterovaginal prolapse
D means emptying the bladder on straining
E is more common in multiparous women

2.75 Stress incontinence can be treated with
A bladder drill
B long term antibiotic therapy
C colposuspension
D anterior colporrhaphy
E Stamey procedure

2.76 Symptoms of detrusor instability include
A urinary incontinence on straining or coughing
B urgency of micturition
C low backache
D insensible incontinence
E urinary frequency

(Answers overleaf)

2.71 A **False** A cystocele is a prolapse of the anterior vaginal
     B **True**   wall containing bladder. Because the urethrovesical
     C **True**   angle is displaced, stress incontinence may occur,
     D **True**   but this is by no means universal and urinary
     E **False** retention may occur. Frequently the patient is
                  asymptomatic. Treatment, when required, is
                  surgical unless there are contraindications.

2.72 A **True**   Asymptomatic bacteriuria is a colony count of
     B **True**   100 000 per ml of urine or more, without symptoms
     C **False** and is usually due to coliforms. It occurs in about
     D **False** 6% of women of reproductive age.
     E **False**

2.73 A **False** Stress incontinence is a mechanical problem
     B **True**   associated with alteration of the urethrovesical
     C **False** angle, particularly with cystoceles, urethroceles or
     D **False** both. Rectoceles do not cause urinary incontinence.
     E **True**   Disseminated sclerosis may present with bladder
                  instability. Patients with myasthenia gravis do not
                  usually complain of urinary symptoms.

2.74 A **True**   Stress incontinence is more common following
     B **False** childbirth. Prolapse does not necessarily cause
     C **False** alteration of the urethrovesical angle and many
     D **False** women with prolapse are not incontinent.
     E **True**   Frequency is a symptom of bladder instability, as is
                  emptying the bladder on straining; in stress
                  incontinence only a few drops are lost on straining.

2.75 A **False** Treatment is repair of the urethrovesical angle by
     B **False** buttressing it upwards by anterior colporrhaphy or
     C **True**   pulling it upwards by colposuspension or sling
     D **True**   procedures.
     E **True**

2.76 A **True**   Detrusor or bladder instability causes urinary
     B **True**   incontinence and frequency. The patient knows that
     C **False** she is about to be incontinent but can do nothing
     D **False** about it. Coughing and raising intra-abdominal
     E **True**   pressure is frequently sufficient stimulus to make
                  the bladder contract.

2.77 Management of a case of chronic bladder instability would usefully include
A   bladder drill
B   anterior colporrhaphy
C   colposuspension
D   cystoscopy
E   oxybutinin

2.78 A vesicovaginal fistula is sometimes a complication of
A   hysterectomy
B   pelvic radiotherapy
C   chronic urinary tract infection
D   advanced cervical carcinoma
E   endometriosis

2.79 Women with urinary incontinence
A   may have a urinary fistula
B   often have a mixed picture of stress and urge incontinence
C   should have an MSU taken
D   should all have bladder pressure studies
E   may be made worse with surgery to the bladder neck

2.80 Backache due to gynaecological causes
A   may be caused by a mobile retroverted uterus
B   is usually felt in the lumbar area
C   may be caused by endometriosis
D   may be due to uterine prolapse
E   may be due to chronic pelvic infection

TUMOURS AND TUMOUR RELATED PROBLEMS

2.81 Pruritus vulvae
A   is commoner in women aged over than under 40 years
B   is also known as vulvodynia
C   may be caused by lichen sclerosus
D   is the commonest presenting symptom in cases of vulval cancer
E   is frequently due to eczema

2.82 Lichen sclerosus
A   leads to vulval cancer in 20% of cases
B   can coexist with VIN
C   is the same as vulval atrophy
D   is best treated by vulvectomy
E   causes disappearance of the contours of the vulva

(Answers overleaf)

2.77 A **True** Bladder instability is not treated surgically.
      B **False** Cystoscopy may be necessary to exclude an
      C **False** intrinsic bladder lesion, but in general bladder drill
      D **True** and anti-cholinergics are the most successful
      E **True** treatments.

2.78 A **True** Vesicovaginal fistulae are uncommon and occur
      B **True** when the pelvic organs have been traumatised,
      C **True** surgically or by radiotherapy, or when a pelvic
      D **True** cancer is present, particularly cervical. The patient
      E **True** with a fistula frequently has all of these factors.

2.79 A **True** Urinary incontinence can be caused by either
      B **True** genuine stress incontinence or detrusor instability.
      C **True** It is rarely caused by a urinary fistula. They should
      D **False** all have an MSU taken and most women should
      E **True** have bladder pressure studies prior to treatment.
                   Most women have a mixed picture of stress and
                   urge incontinence. Some women, however, have
                   clear symptoms and signs of genuine stress
                   incontinence and do not need bladder pressure
                   studies. Many women with detrusor instability will
                   have their symptoms made worse by surgery to the
                   bladder neck.

2.80 A **False** Backache due to gynaecological causes may be due
      B **False** to stretching (prolapse) or irritation (endometriosis,
      C **True** infection) of the uterosacral ligaments and is not
      D **True** caused by mobile retroversion.
      E **True**

TUMOURS AND TUMOUR RELATED PROBLEMS

2.81 A **True** Pruritus vulvae, vulval itching, is most frequently
      B **False** due to eczema or lichen sclerosus. It is commonest
      C **True** after the age of 40 years. Although it may be the
      D **False** presenting complaint of patients with vulval cancer,
      E **True** they usually present with a mass. Vulvodynia is a
                   burning sensation in the vulva and is entirely
                   separate from vulval pruritus.

2.82 A **False** Progressive disease leading to labial adhesions and
      B **True** disappearance of vulval anatomy is the hallmark of
      C **False** lichen sclerosus. Although there is an atrophic
      D **False** element, lichen sclerosus is not pure atrophy and it
      E **True** does not respond to oestrogens. The condition can
                   co-exist with VIN, but has a malignant potential of
                   its own of around 4%. Despite this, local
                   vulvectomy is of no value, the condition frequently
                   returns. Steroids are the treatment of choice.

2.83 Lichen sclerosus

A may affect perianal skin
B is synonymous with leukoplakia
C is associated with autoimmune diseases
D is caused by wart virus infection
E should be treated by laser vaporisation

2.84 Vulval ulceration may be due to

A Crohn's disease
B Behçet's disease
C VIN
D squamous cancer of the vulva
E secondary syphilis

2.85 The following conditions have malignant potential

A vulval intraepithelial neoplasia
B lichen sclerosus
C syphilis
D Paget's disease
E infection with herpes simplex virus 2 (HSV 2)

2.86 Acceptable terms to describe types of vulval disease include

A vulval dystrophy
B squamous cell hyperplasia
C leukoplakia
D Paget's disease
E mixed dystrophy

(Answers overleaf)

2.83 A **True**   Lichen sclerosus affects the vulva and perineum as
      B **False**   well as the perianal area. In approximately 10% of
      C **True**   cases it is associated with autoimmune diseases
      D **False**   such as thyroid problems or pernicious anaemia. It
      E **False**   is not related to wart virus infection. Leukoplakia
                     simply means 'white patch' and could apply to
                     virtually any vulval disease. Laser vaporisation, like
                     vulvectomy, is of no value.

2.84 A **True**   Vulval ulceration is present in approximately 25% of
      B **True**   cases of Crohn's disease in women and may
      C **False**   precede the bowel symptoms. Behçet's disease is a
      D **True**   chronic condition causing oral, genital and ocular
      E **False**   ulceration. VIN does not ulcerate, but invasive
                     cancer may. Primary syphilis will cause ulcers to
                     appear on the vulva but not secondary syphilis.

2.85 A **True**   Both VIN and lichen sclerosus have malignant
      B **True**   potential, estimated as a 4% risk of developing
      C **False**   squamous cancer of the vulva when the condition
      D **True**   is left untreated. Vulval Paget's disease is
      E **False**   associated with a 25% risk of underlying
                     adenocarcinoma developing and is also associated
                     with tumours elsewhere, particularly breast and
                     colon. While development of squamous cancer of
                     the vulva may be associated with the human
                     papilloma (wart) virus infection, there is no
                     evidence to implicate HSV 2. Although early work
                     suggested that syphilis might be an aetiological
                     factor, this has now been discounted and probably
                     reflects coincidental wart virus infection.

2.86 A **False**   The term vulval dystrophy has now been abandoned,
      B **True**   along with the old classification which included mixed
      C **False**   dystrophy. Leukoplakia only means 'white patch',
      D **True**   which could be anything. Vulval skin disease is
      E **False**   described as lichen sclerosus, squamous cell
                     hyperplasia, other dermatoses, VIN (I, II or III) and
                     non-squamous VIN – Paget's disease. If more than
                     one type of disease co-exists with another both are to
                     be listed.

2.87 Vulval intraepithelial neoplasia (VIN)

A is rare in women under 40 years of age
B is not visible to the naked eye
C can be stained with acetic acid
D must be biopsied
E is effectively treated by laser vaporisation

2.88 Paget's disease of the vulva and perineum

A usually presents as a mass
B is associated with cervical malignancy
C is associated with cancers of the large bowel
D is treated by limited local excision
E is treated best by radiotherapy

2.89 Invasive cancer of the vulva

A is usually squamous in type
B carries a poor prognosis
C is best treated by local vulvectomy
D is painful
E is associated with other genital malignancies

2.90 In the staging of vulval cancers

A stage II lesions are confined to the vulva and perineum
B stage I lesions are microinvasive
C bilateral groin node involvement puts the patient in stage IV
D involvement of the anus puts the patient in stage III
E involvement of the vagina is stage IV disease

(Answers overleaf)

2.87 A **False**   40% of women with VIN are aged under 40. The
    B **False**   lesions are often raised and roughened and may be
    C **True**   white or red. They can usually be seen with the naked
    D **True**   eye but do become more apparent with 5% acetic acid
    E **False**   staining. Biopsy is essential to establish the diagnosis
and to exclude malignancy in suspicious areas.
Treatment is difficult, and laser vaporisation has
proved disappointing. Recurrence rates for this form
of treatment are the same as after vulvectomy, up to
45%.

2.88 A **False**   Paget's disease usually presents with pruritus
    B **True**   vulvae. It is associated with an underlying
    C **True**   adenocarcinoma in 25% of cases, but concomitant
    D **False**   genital malignancy is also frequently seen,
    E **False**   especially in the cervix. If Paget's involves the anal
canal, as it frequently does, there is a 70% risk of
colonic or rectal cancers developing. Treatment is
by wide local excision as the lesion frequently
extends further than the apparent skin lesion.
Treatment with retinoids may also help.

2.89 A **True**   Approximately 90% of vulval cancers are squamous,
    B **False**   the next commonest being malignant melanoma. The
    C **False**   condition generally carries a good prognosis, stages I
    D **False**   and II having more than 70% five-year survival and
    E **True**   even stage III having a five-year survival around 40%.
Treatment is with radical surgery and bilateral groin
node dissection as even small tumours may have
metastasised to lymph nodes. Pain is a late and
uncommon complaint. Co-existing genital cancer or
pre-malignant disease is seen, especially in the
cervix, in a significant proportion of cases and should
always be sought for.

2.90 A **True**   Stage I and stage II cancer of the vulva are both
    B **False**   confined to the vulva and perineum, stage I lesions
    C **True**   being less than 2 cm in diameter. A true microinvasive
    D **True**   stage does not exist. Local spread to the urethra,
    E **False**   vagina or anus and metastasis to ipsilateral groin
lymph nodes are all stage III disease. Bilateral groin
node involvement or more extensive spread put the
patient in stage IV.

2.91 Vaginal intraepithelial neoplasia (VAIN)
A   is usually associated with CIN
B   is a superficial condition
C   occurring after hysterectomy, is best treated by laser
    vaporisation
D   is effectively treated by radiation
E   has colposcopic appearances similar to those of CIN

2.92 Primary carcinoma of the vagina
A   is usually an adenocarcinoma
B   is usually treated with radiotherapy
C   more commonly occurs in the upper vagina than in the
    lower
D   usually presents as pelvic pain
E   is associated with cervical cancer

2.93 Indications for cone biopsy include
A   a visible squamo-columnar junction
B   suspicion of invasive malignancy
C   glandular atypicalities in the cervical smear
D   severe dyskaryosis in the cervical smear
E   an abnormal smear in a patient who has previously been
    treated for a cervical lesion

**2.94 In assessing the histological type of cervical intraepithelial
neoplasia (CIN) present, the following factors are taken into
account**
A   the presence of human papilloma virus (HPV)
B   numbers of mitotic figures
C   the nuclear-cytoplasmic ratio
D   epithelial differentiation
E   crypt involvement

2.95 Adenocarcinoma in situ of the cervix (AIS)
A   is diagnosed by cervical cytology
B   is detected by cervical cytology
C   is frequently associated with CIN
D   is usually diagnosed at colposcopy
E   usually lies high in the canal away from the
    squamo-columnar junction

(Answers overleaf)

2.91 A   **True**   Isolated VAIN is uncommon, usually it is an extension
      B   **True**   of CIN onto the vagina. Because there are no crypts in
      C   **False**   the vagina the disease is superficial. After
      D   **True**   hysterectomy, abnormal areas may be buried in the
      E   **True**   suture line and radiotherapy or surgical removal of
the vault is necessary. The colposcopic appearances
are similar to those seen on the cervix, although they
can be more difficult to evaluate.

2.92 A   **False**   Primary cancer of the vagina is usually squamous
      B   **True**   (90%). It is best treated with radiotherapy, although
      C   **True**   stage I lesions of the upper vagina can be treated
      D   **False**   by Wertheim's hysterectomy. The upper vagina is
      E   **False**   the commonest site. Pelvic pain is an uncommon
presenting symptom. If cervical cancer is present it
is assumed that the vaginal lesion is secondary to it
and not a primary.

2.93 A   **False**   Indications for cone biopsy include an inability to
      B   **True**   see the squamo-columnar junction, suspicion of
      C   **True**   invasion or microinvasion, extension of the
      D   **False**   abnormal area high into the cervical canal and the
      E   **True**   presence of glandular abnormalities in the smear. If
a patient has previously been treated for a cervical
lesion, the anatomy of the squamo-columnar
junction and transformation zone has been
distorted and there may be satellite lesions in the
canal; cone biopsy is indicated. Severe dyskaryosis
is an indication for colposcopy.

2.94 A   **False**   HPV is frequently associated with CIN and may
      B   **True**   have a causal role, but it does not help to
      C   **True**   differentiate between the various grades. Neither
      D   **True**   does crypt involvement, which may be present at
      E   **False**   any grade. The larger the number of mitotic figures,
the greater the nuclear-cytoplasmic ratio and the
poorer the epithelial differentiation, especially as
these factors near the epithelial surface, the worse
the grade (i.e. the more likely it is to be CIN III than
CIN I).

2.95 A   **False**   Glandular abnormalities associated with AIS can be
      B   **True**   detected by cervical cytology, but the diagnosis
      C   **True**   depends upon histology. CIN and AIS frequently
      D   **False**   co-exist. AIS is usually diagnosed at cone biopsy or
      E   **False**   hysterectomy. Most of the lesions are very close, or
adjacent to the squamo-columnar junction.

2.96 When using exfoliative cytology to diagnose cervical neoplasia

A the aim is to sample the surface cells of the cervical transformation zone
B the sampling device must cover 360° of the cervix
C aspiration of cells from the posterior fornix pool is as useful as using an Ayre spatula to scrape the cervical surface
D the presence of endometrial cancer will be detected in 70% of cases
E fixation must take place immediately

2.97 CIN III lesions extending into the cervical canal are

A often invasive
B treated by radiotherapy
C treated by hysterectomy
D safely treated by cone biopsy
E safely treated by large loop excision of the transformation zone

2.98 Cervical intraepithelial neoplasia (CIN)

A may present with postcoital bleeding
B may present with intermenstrual bleeding
C is also known as an ectropion
D is usually asymptomatic
E presents with a vaginal discharge

2.99 In a patient who is 12 weeks pregnant, severe atypicalities in a cervical smear indicate a need for

A colposcopy
B a repeat cervical smear
C termination of pregnancy
D cone biopsy
E random punch biopsy of the cervix

(Answers overleaf)

2.96 A **True** The cervical transformation zone is the site of
B **True** development of CIN lesions. Because the lesions may
C **False** be small, the whole area must be scraped. Sampling
D **False** cells from the posterior fornix has an unacceptably
E **True** high false negative rate. Endometrial cancer is
diagnosed in only 25% of cases. If fixation does not
take place immediately, drying artefacts occur in the
smear which make it difficult to interpret.

2.97 A **False** CIN III lesions are not invasive, and treatment by
B **False** radiotherapy or hysterectomy is not necessary. As the
C **False** lesion extends into the canal it cannot be guaranteed
D **True** that the worst part has been seen at colposcopy, so
E **True** biopsy of the area that can be seen is not helpful.
Cone biopsy is required, or alternatively, large loop
excision of the transformation zone. These
procedures provide specimens which can be
assessed histologically so that the diagnosis can be
arrived at. In most cases, removal of the lesion at
cone biopsy or loop excision is also curative.

2.98 A **False** Cervical intraepithelial neoplasia does not cause
B **False** any symptoms and the lesion can usually not be
C **False** seen by the naked eye. Cervical ectropion is an
D **True** eversion of the columnar epithelium so that it is
E **False** visible on the vaginal portion of the cervix. The
presence of postcoital or intermenstrual bleeding or
a vaginal discharge when the cervical smear is
abnormal is either coincidental or is suspicious of
invasive cancer of the cervix.

2.99 A **True** Severe atypicalities appearing in a cervical smear in
B **True** pregnancy indicate a need for colposcopy. Although it
C **False** might be argued that the smear should be repeated,
D **False** this generally just wastes time if the atypicalities are
E **False** severe. These lesions can progress rapidly and
colposcopic review may be necessary again later in
pregnancy. Termination of pregnancy would only be
considered if invasive cancer was present. Punch
biopsy is only of use when a lesion can be seen, never
randomly. Cone biopsy is avoided in pregnancy if at
all possible because of the risk of haemorrhage.

2.100 Apparent incomplete excision of CIN at cone biopsy is best managed initially by

A   abdominal hysterectomy when CIN extends to the endocervical limit of the cone

B   vaginal hysterectomy when the CIN extends to the ectocervical limit of the cone

C   radiotherapy

D   repeat cone biopsy

E   follow up cytology

2.101 Invasive cancer of the cervix

A   is the commonest malignant tumour in women in the United Kingdom

B   occurs most commonly in women under the age of 40 years

C   is usually of squamous type

D   occurs more commonly in women who smoke cigarettes

E   is uncommon in developing countries

2.102 Microinvasive cancer of the cervix

A   consists only of those showing early stromal invasion

B   may invade to a depth of 5 mm

C   should have a maximum width of 7 mm

D   may invade lymphatic channels

E   have not metastasised

2.103 In stage II carcinoma of the cervix

A   the growth is confined to the cervix

B   there may be extension into the body of the uterus

C   the upper third of the vagina may be involved

D   the tumour is fixed to the lateral pelvic wall

E   a five-year survival rate of 80% can be expected

(Answers overleaf)

2.100 A **False**   In the vast majority of cases in which CIN extends
      B **False**   to the limits of excision on a cone biopsy no
      C **False**   residual CIN is present in the remaining cervix. In
      D **False**   the past, hysterectomies performed on these
      E **True**   patients showed no residual disease in most cases
and it is not now thought necessary to recommend
hysterectomy, abdominal or vaginal, as the initial
treatment. Similarly, neither radiotherapy nor repeat
cone biopsy are necessary. The patient should be
subjected to follow up cytology, with or without
colposcopy, and only if there is a demonstrable
abnormality on the cervix should further treatment
be undertaken.

2.101 A **False**   Invasive cancer of the cervix accounts for 4% of
      B **False**   malignancies in women in the United Kingdom. The
      C **True**   commonest tumours are of breast and lung.
      D **True**   However, in the world as a whole, cancer of the
      E **False**   cervix is second only to breast cancer. The disease
is becoming commoner in young women, but the
peak age is still between 55 and 60 years. More
than 85% of these tumours are squamous in type,
but adenocarcinoma is becoming more common,
particularly in younger women. There is a strong
epidemiological link with smoking cigarettes.

2.102 A **False**   Early stromal invasion is the earliest recognisable
      B **True**   stage of invasion. Minute areas of malignant cells
      C **True**   push through the basement membrane into the
      D **True**   cervical stroma. Microinvasive carcinoma is defined
      E **False**   as a lesion which has a maximum depth of invasion
of not more than 5 mm and a maximum width of
not more 7 mm. Lymphatic channels may be
involved. Unfortunately, this definition is not
particularly useful as the larger microinvasive
lesions may have already metastasised to regional
lymph nodes in which case local treatment, such as
cone biopsy, is no longer appropriate.

2.103 A **False**   In stage I the growth is confined to the cervix. In stage
      B **True**   IIa the upper two-thirds of the vagina may be
      C **True**   involved and in IIb the tumour extends into the
      D **False**   parametrium, but only becomes fixed to the pelvic
      E **False**   side wall in stage III. The staging is performed at
examination under anaesthetic. Extension into the
body of the uterus cannot be detected at bimanual
examination and does not feature in the staging. As it
does not alter the prognosis this does not matter. A
five-year survival rate of approximately 60% can be
expected.

2.104 In the United Kingdom the common presentations of carcinoma of the cervix are

A   an asymptomatic abnormal smear
B   pelvic pain
C   vaginal discharge
D   postcoital bleeding
E   intermenstrual bleeding

2.105 The following investigations are necessary for adequate staging of cancer of the cervix

A   a vaginal examination under anaesthetic
B   cystoscopy
C   lymph node biopsy
D   lymphangiography
E   rectal examination under anaesthetic

2.106 Carcinoma of the endometrium

A   occurs at a median age of approximately 60 years
B   is most common in postmenopausal women
C   is exceptionally rare in women under the age of 40 years
D   is more common in grand multipara than nullipara
E   is less common in the United Kingdom than in developing countries

2.107 Postmenopausal bleeding is a common presentation of

A   cervical ectropion
B   carcinoma of the endometrium
C   atrophic vaginitis
D   carcinoma of the cervix
E   uterine fibroids

(Answers overleaf)

2.104 A **True**   Classically invasive cancer of the cervix presents
      B **False** with postcoital or intermenstrual bleeding or an
      C **True**   offensive vaginal discharge. Pain is an uncommon
      D **True**   and late phenomenon. Increasingly, patients are
      E **True**   presenting without symptoms having had a routine
               cervical smear.

2.105 A **True**   The staging of cancer of the cervix is performed at
      B **True**   examination under anaesthetic. Bimanual
      C **False** examination may reveal the tumour on the cervix
      D **False** with or without extension into the vagina and the
      E **True**   parametrium. Extension into the parametrium is
               more easily felt on rectal examination under
               anaesthetic. Extension into the mucosa of the
               bladder is seen at cystoscopy. Involvement of
               lymph nodes does not affect the staging so neither
               lymph node biopsy nor lymphangiography are of
               value.

2.106 A **True**   Endometrial cancer is mainly a disease of the
      B **True**   postmenopausal woman. Approximately 80% are
      C **False** postmenopausal, although up to 5% will occur in
      D **False** women under the age of 40 years. Nullipara are at
      E **False** considerably more risk than parous women, and
               this accounts for some of the geographical
               differences, the highest rates being in North
               America and Western Europe, the lowest in
               developing countries.

2.107 A **False** Patients presenting with postmenopausal bleeding
      B **True**   should always be investigated because it is the
      C **True**   commonest presentation of early endometrial
      D **True**   cancer. Despite the increase in cervical cancer in
      E **False** younger women, many cervical cancers are
               diagnosed in postmenopausal women, and in these
               cases the presentation is often postmenopausal
               bleeding. The commonest cause of postmenopausal
               bleeding is atrophic vaginitis (although problems
               with hormone replacement therapy may overtake
               it). A diagnosis of cervical ectropion (a hormonal
               event) is difficult to sustain after the menopause.
               Fibroids get smaller after the menopause, and with
               the exception of fibroid polyps, which are
               uncommon, do not cause symptoms at this stage
               of life.

2.108 The following factors increase the risk of a woman developing endometrial cancer

A obesity
B early menopause
C combined (oestrogen and progestogen) hormone replacement therapy
D diabetes mellitus
E a history of polycystic ovary disease

2.109 Endometrial adenocarcinomas

A are derived from endometrial stroma
B may include areas of benign squamous epithelium
C may include areas of malignant squamous epithelium
D are the commonest tumours of the endometrium
E contain malignant glands and stroma

2.110 In patients with endometrial adenocarcinoma the following factors improve the prognosis

A a history of anovulatory infertility
B a history of taking oestrogen only hormone replacement therapy
C increasing age
D benign squamous elements in the tumour
E superficial myometrial invasion

2.111 The following statements concerning endometrial cancer are correct

A involvement of the cervix occurs in stage II disease
B invasion of the myometrium to a depth of more than 50% puts the case into stage II
C initial treatment of stage I disease is by total abdominal hysterectomy and bilateral salpingo-oophorectomy
D postoperative radiotherapy is rarely required in stage I disease
E five-year survival is 90%

(Answers overleaf)

2.108   A **True**   Oestrogenic stimulation of the endometrium leads
        B **False**   to proliferation and, if continued unopposed for
        C **False**   long enough, atypicalities and eventually cancer. In
        D **True**   postmenopausal women the major oestrogen is
        E **True**   oestrone which is partly derived from androgens by
                       aromatisation in adipose tissue. The effect of
                       diabetes mellitus may be related to increased
                       weight. In polycystic ovary disease there is an
                       excess of oestrogens. Treatment with combined
                       hormone replacement therapy protects against
                       cancer of the endometrium, causing reduced
                       proliferation and regular shedding at menstruation.
                       Late menopause is associated with development of
                       endometrial cancer.

2.109   A **False**   Endometrial adenocarcinoma, the commonest
        B **True**   malignancy of the body of the uterus, is derived
        C **True**   from the glandular elements of the endometrium.
        D **True**   Sarcomas are derived from the stromal elements. In
        E **False**   as many as 25% of cases squamous elements are
                       seen, either benign or malignant. The combination
                       of malignant glandular and stromal elements lead
                       to the uncommon diagnosis of mixed Mullerian
                       tumour.

2.110   A **True**   Patients who have developed endometrial carcinoma
        B **True**   because of oestrogenic stimulation are more likely to
        C **False**   have well differentiated tumours with a good
        D **True**   prognosis. These include patients with histories of
        E **True**   anovulatory infertility and oestrogen only hormone
                       replacement therapy. Younger women have a better
                       prognosis than older. Benign squamous elements
                       confer a good prognosis, but if the squamous
                       elements are malignant the prognosis is worse than
                       adenocarcinoma alone. Depth of invasion is one of
                       the best prognostic indicators, superficial being much
                       better than deep invasion.

2.111   A **True**   Stage I disease is confined to the body of the
        B **False**   uterus, including myometrial invasion (not
        C **True**   penetration) to any depth. The cervix is involved in
        D **False**   stage II disease and this carries a worse prognosis.
        E **False**   Initial treatment of stage I disease is total
                       abdominal hysterectomy and bilateral salpingo-
                       oophorectomy, with or without pelvic node
                       dissection. In poorly differentiated cases, or when
                       the myometrium is invaded more than superficially,
                       radiotherapy is required. The overall five-year
                       survival (all cases) is approximately 65%.

2.112 Uterine fibroids

    A originate from smooth muscle
    B contain muscle and connective tissues
    C are usually multiple
    D are usually submucous
    E are uncommon in the cervix

2.113 Fibroids

    A are oestrogen dependent
    B get smaller during treatment with progestogens
    C are usually asymptomatic
    D shrink in response to treatment with LHRH agonists
    E are very vascular

2.114 Intramural fibroids cause

    A intermenstrual bleeding
    B postcoital bleeding
    C postmenopausal bleeding
    D deep dyspareunia
    E polymenorrhoea

2.115 Endometrial polyps

    A occur most frequently in postmenopausal women
    B cause intermenstrual bleeding
    C have increased malignant potential
    D are treated by hysterectomy
    E may present as dysmenorrhoea

(Answers overleaf)

2.112 A **True**   Although called fibroids, these tumours are derived
      B **True**   from smooth muscle and are really leiomyomata.
      C **True**   Fibroids contain smooth muscle and variable
      D **False**   amounts of connective tissue and are usually
      E **True**   multiple. They may be subserous, intramural and in
                    only 5% of cases submucous. Fibroids can occur in
                    the cervix but are relatively uncommon.

2.113 A **True**   Fibroids occur in reproductive age and get smaller
      B **False**   after the menopause. They may enlarge in high
      C **True**   oestrogenic states such as pregnancy but certainly
      D **True**   get smaller in artificial hypo-oestrogenic states such
      E **False**   as treatment with LHRH agonists. The effect of
                    progesterone is uncertain, but they do not get smaller
                    when the patient is treated with progestogens.
                    Fibroids are very common and often asymptomatic.
                    Although the vascularity of the uterus is increased,
                    the fibroids themselves are relatively avascular.

2.114 A **False**   The major problem with fibroids is that they are
      B **False**   common and all of a woman's gynaecological
      C **False**   symptoms may be ascribed to them. Whilst
      D **False**   submucous fibroids or fibroid polyps may become
      E **False**   eroded and cause intermenstrual or postcoital
                    bleeding, that is not true of intramural fibroids. In
                    general, fibroids do not cause problems after the
                    menopause. Pain is uncommon; there may be clot
                    colic in menorrhagia or the pain of red degeneration
                    (most common in pregnancy) but deep dyspareunia
                    is unlikely. Fibroids cause menorrhagia and do not
                    generally affect cycle length.

2.115 A **False**   Endometrial polyps occur most frequently in the
      B **True**   decade before the menopause. The endometrial
      C **False**   surface of the polyp frequently becomes eroded and
      D **False**   may cause intermenstrual bleeding or even postcoital
      E **True**   bleeding. There is no increase in the malignant
                    potential of the epithelium of a polyp compared with
                    epithelium elsewhere in the uterus and treatment is
                    removal at curettage rather than hysterectomy. If the
                    polyp is large the uterus may attempt to expel it and
                    this may cause dysmenorrhoea.

2.116 The following factors increase the risk of a woman developing ovarian cancer

A multiparity
B use of an oral contraceptive
C having a family history of ovarian cancer
D late age at menarche
E superovulation

2.117 The following are types of epithelial ovarian tumours

A endometrioid adenocarcinoma
B transitional cell tumour
C dysgerminoma
D thecoma
E mucinous cystadenocarcinoma

2.118 Fibromas of the ovary

A frequently become malignant
B may be associated with ascites
C often contain teeth
D may be associated with a hydrothorax
E commonly present as a large abdominal mass

2.119 Common sites for tumours metastasising to the ovary are

A stomach
B lung
C colon
D breast
E oesophagus

2.120 The following tumours of the ovary are commonly hormone secreting

A granulosa cell
B Leydig cell tumours
C benign cystic teratomas
D transitional cell tumours
E serous cystadenomas

(Answers overleaf)

2.116   A   **False**   There is clear evidence of decreasing risk of
        B   **False**   developing ovarian cancer with increasing parity.
        C   **True**   Active ovulation is thought to be a major
        D   **False**   aetiological factor and use of ovulation suppressing
        E   **True**   oral contraceptives reduces the risk. Similarly, it
                        might be thought that early menarche and late
                        menopause would increase the risk, but this is
                        unclear. Although the risk increases with years of
                        ovulation, anovulatory cycles are so frequent to the
                        extremes of reproductive life that timing of
                        menarche and menopause has no clear effect.
                        There is a strong genetic component and females
                        with affected first degree relatives are at significant
                        risk. Recent reports of the occurrence of carcinoma
                        in patients on infertility programmes have
                        supported the theory that repeated superovulation
                        induces malignant change in the ovary.

2.117   A   **True**   Epithelial ovarian tumours include benign and
        B   **True**   malignant forms of endometrioid, serous and
        C   **False**   mucinous tumours and transitional cell (Brenner)
        D   **False**   tumours. Dysgerminomas are germ cell tumours.
        E   **True**

2.118   A   **False**   Ovarian fibromas are sex cord tumours which are
        B   **True**   invariably benign. Ascites is found in 20–30% of
        C   **False**   cases, and in Meigs syndrome. This is associated
        D   **True**   with hydrothorax (1% of cases). They are of
        E   **False**   variable size, mostly presenting as moderate sized
                        asymptomatic pelvic, rather than abdominal
                        masses. Teratomas not fibromas contain teeth.

2.119   A   **True**   The ovaries are a common site for secondary
        B   **True**   deposits from primaries elsewhere, particularly
        C   **True**   from the breast, stomach and colon. They also
        D   **False**   become involved by tumours that become widely
        E   **False**   disseminated such as malignant melanomas and
                        lymphomas.

2.120   A   **True**   Granulosa cell tumours commonly secrete
        B   **True**   oestrogens, as do theca cell tumours. Oestrogen
        C   **False**   production can cause endometrial hyperplasia and
        D   **False**   in approximately 6% of cases co-existing
        E   **False**   endometrial adenocarcinoma may be found. Leydig
                        cell tumours produce androgens and lead to
                        virilism.

2.121 Spread of epithelial ovarian cancers

  A via the blood stream occurs early in the disease
  B to para-aortic lymph nodes puts the case at stage III
  C to the underside of the diaphragm is common
  D around the peritoneal cavity has usually occurred by the time of diagnosis
  E to the omentum frequently occurs

2.122 Frequently seen symptoms of ovarian malignancy include

  A abdominal distension
  B sharp, severe pelvic pain
  C bloating and nausea
  D abnormal uterine bleeding
  E breathlessness

2.123 The following tumour markers are correctly linked with the tumours that secrete them

  A human chorionic gonadotrophin: ovarian choriocarcinoma
  B alphafetoprotein: endodermal sinus tumour
  C CA125: dysgerminoma
  D oestrogens: granulosa cell tumours
  E testosterone: theca cell tumours

2.124 Dysgerminomas

  A are bilateral in 50% of cases
  B are commoner in younger than older women
  C frequently present with abdominal pain
  D are common in patients with testicular feminisation syndrome
  E are treated initially by radiotherapy

2.125 Chemotherapeutic agents used to treat epithelial ovarian cancers

  A usually effect a cure
  B should contain platinum for best effect
  C are best given continually for six months
  D should be used for all stages of the disease
  E are more effective after cytoreductive surgery

(Answers overleaf)

2.121 A **False** Most ovarian cancers present late when the patient
      B **True**   is already at least stage III. Spread has usually
      C **True**   occurred transcoelomically to the omentum and the
      D **True**   peritoneum, particularly under the diaphragm. In
      E **True**   stage III, tumour is limited to the peritoneal cavity
                   and pelvic organs and to retroperitoneal nodes.
                   Haematogenous spread is late.

2.122 A **True**   Characteristically ovarian cancers develop silently
      B **False** or with vague symptoms of discomfort and
      C **True**   abdominal swelling. Sharp pain is uncommon.
      D **True**   Although abnormal uterine bleeding is mainly
      E **False** associated with oestrogen secreting tumours such
                   as granulosa cell tumour, it frequently occurs in
                   epithelial tumours as well (some of these may be
                   oestrogen secreting). Breathlessness is only a
                   feature when there is a large pleural effusion.

2.123 A **True**   Tumour markers may be of value in reaching a
      B **True**   diagnosis before operation, but are of most value in
      C **False** evaluating treatment and in follow up. HCG is
      D **True**   produced by trophoblast and ovarian
      E **False** choriocarcinoma. Alphafetoprotein is produced by
                   two-thirds of germ cell tumours, particularly when
                   they are not poorly differentiated. Hormone
                   secreting tumours such as granulosa cell and theca
                   cell tumours produce oestrogens. Sertoli–Leydig
                   cell tumours may produce testosterone.

2.124 A **False** Dysgerminomas are bilateral in 10–15% of cases.
      B **True**   They generally occur in girls and young women.
      C **True**   Abdominal pain is common, is present in over 80%
      D **True**   of cases and is severe in 10%. If a Y chromosome is
      E **False** present in a phenotypic female the risk of germ cell
                   tumour occurring, usually dysgerminoma, is about
                   25%. Initial treatment is surgical. In young women,
                   fertility can frequently be preserved, even after
                   treatment with chemotherapy as well as surgery.

2.125 A **False** Chemotherapy for ovarian cancer rarely cures the
      B **True**   patient in current practice. Platinum containing
      C **False** drugs, either alone or in combination with
      D **False** alkylating agents, appear to be the most effective in
      E **True**   obtaining and maintaining a response. They are
                   usually given once a month, allowing time for
                   recovery from toxicity between courses.
                   Chemotherapy is not necessary in stage Ia disease
                   and possibly not in Ib or Ic as well. The smaller the
                   quantity of residual tumour the more effective the
                   chemotherapeutic agent is likely to be.

INFERTILITY AND SOCIAL GYNAECOLOGY

2.126 Azoospermic males
A   do not ejaculate
B   should have a serum FSH performed
C   usually have a low serum testosterone concentration
D   can sometimes father children
E   commonly have a chromosomal abnormality

2.127 Oligozoospermia
A   is defined as a sperm density of less of 5 000 000 per ml
B   usually responds well to a three-month course of clomiphene citrate
C   is associated with cryptorchidism
D   would make it unlikely that a man would father a child
E   may be caused by high scrotal temperature

2.128 A normal semen sample should
A   contain white blood cells
B   liquefy within 30 minutes
C   have a volume of more than 4 ml
D   have a sperm count of more than 20 000 000 per ml
E   have at least 60% sperm motility, 30 minutes after production

2.129 Women with anovulatory subfertility
A   usually have a 28-day menstrual cycle
B   usually have an elevated FSH level
C   should have an ovarian biopsy
D   should have a serum prolactin estimation
E   if they are amenorrhoeic should have a progesterone challenge test

(Answers overleaf)

INFERTILITY AND SOCIAL GYNAECOLOGY

2.126 A **False**   Azoospermic males have no sperm within a normal
       B **True**   ejaculate. If there is no ejaculate*then retrograde
       C **False**   ejaculation must be ruled out. Only one in 20
       D **True**   azoospermic men have a chromosomal abnormality.
       E **False**   Most men have seminiferous tubular failure and
therefore have elevated serum FSH concentrations.
Leydig cell function, however, continues normally and
most men have normal LH and testosterone
concentrations. If the serum FSH level is normal, then
obstruction or congenital absence of the vas must be
excluded by testicular biopsy and vasography. If
sperm are being produced but are not appearing in
the ejaculate then modern techniques like testicular
or epididymal aspiration or microsurgery of the vas
can sometimes allow these men to father children.

2.127 A **False**   Oligozoospermia is usually defined as a sperm
       B **False**   density of less than 20 000 000 per ml. Drug
       C **True**   treatment of oligozoospermia by clomiphene
       D **False**   citrate, gonadotrophins or androgens only rarely
       E **True**   have a beneficial effect. Spermatogenesis is
prevented by high scrotal temperatures and it is
presumed that this is the reason that boys with
cryptorchidism will often have oligozoospermia in
later life. Many men with oligozoospermia have no
difficulty fathering a child.

2.128 A **False**   A normal semen specimen has a volume of more
       B **True**   than 2 ml with a count of at least 20 000 000 per ml
       C **False**   with more than 60% motility and 60% normal
       D **True**   forms. Liquefaction takes place within 30 minutes.
       E **True**   White cells indicate an infection and the specimen
should be sent for culture and sensitivity. There is a
wide variation in normal semen samples and they
do not test the fertilising capacity of sperm. A low
specimen should always be repeated after three
months and the man should be examined.

2.129 A **False**   Most women with a 28-day cycle ovulate normally
       B **False**   and most women with anovulatory cycles have
       C **False**   oligomenorrhoea. Women with an elevated FSH
       D **True**   level have some degree of ovarian resistance, or
       E **True**   premature menopause. An ovarian biopsy should
only be perfomed to differentiate resistant ovarian
syndrome from premature menopause. All
anovulatory women should have a serum prolactin
estimation. If they are amenorrhoeic a progesterone
challenge test will give a reasonable idea as to
whether anti-oestrogens, e.g. clomiphene citrate,
will be effective in ovulation induction.

2.130 **In the initial investigation of primary subfertility**
A ovulation should be monitored by serial follicular scanning
B a single semen analysis should be analysed
C a hysterosalpingogram is the most appropriate investigation to assess tubal function
D assessment of cervical mucus should only be performed once ovulation has been confirmed
E a basal body temperature chart is essential

2.131 **In secondary infertility**
A the condition is frequently due to tubal problems
B infertility is secondary to some reversible factors
C no living children have been produced by the woman
D the problem is often a chromosomal defect in the woman
E the problem can be one of anovulation

2.132 **A postcoital test**
A should be performed at mid-cycle
B may reveal cervical infection as a cause of infertility
C is positive if no motile sperm are seen in the vaginal secretion
D reliably diagnoses azoospermia
E should be replaced by a sperm invasion test

2.133 **Ovulation can be diagnosed by**
A measuring a day 14 serum progesterone
B observing a rise in basal body temperature in the second half of the menstrual cycle
C study of the cervical mucus
D endometrial biopsy
E a day 21 serum prolactin estimation

(Answers overleaf)

2.130   A   **False**   The initial investigation of primary subfertility may
       B   **False**   include a basal body temperature chart as an
       C   **False**   assessment of ovulation. It is certainly not essential
       D   **True**   and many women find keeping a basal body
       E   **False**   temperature chart unnecessarily invasive on their
lives. In a woman with a regular cycle the easiest
way to assess ovulation is with a mid-luteal
progesterone estimation. Follicular scanning as an
initial investigation is unnecessary and expensive.
Usually two semen analyses should be analysed as
fluctuations can be marked. A laparoscopy and dye
insufflation generally gives more information than a
hysterosalpingogram in terms of tubal function.

2.131   A   **True**   A patient with secondary infertility has been
       B   **False**   pregnant before, whatever the outcome. The
       C   **False**   problem may be due to anovulation, but is more
       D   **False**   frequently due to tubal obstruction secondary to
       E   **True**   infection. Chromosomal defects usually cause
primary amenorrhoea.

2.132   A   **True**   A postcoital test must be performed around the time
       B   **True**   of ovulation. The cervical mucus is viewed following
       C   **False**   intercourse to see if sperm have entered the mucus
       D   **False**   and remain motile within it. Pus cells suggest
       E   **True**   infection and commonly infection will inhibit sperm
motility. Absence of sperm may be due to failure to
enter the mucus, or inadequate intercourse as well as
azoospermia. A crossed sperm invasion test will more
accurately diagnose cervical mucus hostility.

2.133   A   **False**   Detection of ovulation usually depends upon the
       B   **True**   appearance of progesterone after ovulation. The
       C   **True**   hormone causes the patient's temperature to rise
       D   **True**   and the serum concentration should be measured
       E   **False**   in the mid-luteal phase, i.e. between the 19th and
21st days of a 28-day cycle. It causes the
endometrium to develop secretory changes and a
mid-luteal endometrial biopsy can make this
diagnosis. Prolactin concentrations are not reliably
affected by ovulation. The cervical mucus becomes
thinner and more elastic under the influence of
oestrogen at ovulation and shows 'ferning'.

2.134 Primary subfertility
- A should be investigated after six months duration
- B is commonly associated with a male factor
- C is unexplained in about 25% of cases
- D affects about 1 in 10 couples
- E should initially be investigated by the general practitioner

2.135 In vitro fertilisation
- A should have an overall pregnancy rate of about 20% per cycle
- B there is an increased risk of ectopic pregnancy
- C the success rate is lowered if the woman is over 35 years of age
- D is successful treatment for severe oligo-asthenospermia
- E four embryos are usually replaced into the uterine cavity

2.136 Donor insemination (DI)
- A is licensed by the HFEA
- B can be performed for lesbian women
- C is usually performed intravaginally
- D should be continued for at least 24 cycles if the couple are unsuccessful
- E should be combined with ovulation monitoring

2.137 Intrauterine insemination (IUI) is
- A successful treatment for severe male factor subfertility
- B more successful if gonadotrophins are used for ovulation induction
- C requires an anaesthetic
- D requires normal fallopian tubes
- E is as successful as gamete intrafallopian transfer

(Answers overleaf)

2.134 A **False**   Couples who have tried for a pregnancy for six
       B **True**   months still have a high chance of spontaneous
       C **True**   conception and should not generally be investigated
       D **True**   at that time. About 30% of primary subfertility is
       E **True**   associated with a male factor problem and about 25%
                       have an unexplained problem. Subfertility affects
                       about 1 in 10 couples in the United Kingdom at the
                       present time. Initial investigation and even some
                       treatments are ideally suited to general practice.
                       Many infertility units are developing infertility
                       protocols with their local general practitioners.

2.135 A **True**   Most IVF units should expect to have a pregnancy
       B **True**   rate of about 20% per cycle. There is a risk of an
       C **True**   ectopic pregnancy rate of about 5% of cases. The
       D **False**   success rate is lowered by several factors and
       E **False**   maternal age over 35 years is one of these. A total
                       motile count of less than 5 000 000 sperm will give
                       a high chance of failed fertilisation and so it is
                       unlikely that successful treatment will occur. Under
                       the HFEA regulations only three embryos are
                       allowed to be replaced into the uterine cavity
                       following fertilisation. Any spare embryos would be
                       frozen if the IVF unit has cryopreservation facilities.

2.136 A **True**   DI is usually performed into the cervix with
       B **True**   unwashed sperm or into the uterus with washed
       C **False**   sperm. With intrauterine insemination conception
       D **False**   will often occur within four cycles and into the
       E **True**   cervix in about eight cycles. Treatment, therefore,
                       should generally not be continued for 24 cycles.
                       Alternative treatments like IVF using donor sperm
                       should be sought prior to this. In order to be
                       effective DI has to be combined with monitoring of
                       ovulation. Storage and treatment with human
                       gametes is licensed by the HFEA.

2.137 A **False**   Intrauterine insemination involves the preparation
       B **True**   of a sperm sample either using a swim up
       C **False**   technique or through a percol gradient. The sperm
       D **True**   is then passed through a catheter with a syringe
       E **False**   into the uterine cavity. The fallopian tubes must be
                       normal for this technique to be successful, it does
                       not require an anaesthetic and the timing to
                       ovulation is vital. It has a poor success rate in
                       severe male factor subfertility. Success rates with
                       intrauterine insemination increase with ovulation
                       induction and the results with gonadotrophins are
                       better than the result with clomiphene. Pregnancy
                       rates per cycle are still lower than with GIFT.

2.138 In IVF
A superovulation is usually performed using clomiphene and pergonal
B the multiple pregnancy rate increases as the number of embryos replaced increases
C oocyte retrieval is usually performed laparoscopically
D embryo freezing facilities should be available in all units
E donor eggs should be used over the age of 40

2.139 Induction of ovulation may be achieved by giving
A clomiphene citrate
B cyproterone acetate
C progesterone
D FSH and LH
E tamoxifen

2.140 Depo medroxyprogesterone acetate (Depo-Provera)
A needs to be administered intramuscularly every three months to be effective
B is a very effective form of contraception
C rarely has side effects
D fertility may be only slowly resumed
E should not be used in women over 40

2.141 Condoms (the sheath)
A are available free of charge from general practitioners
B should be applied just before ejaculation
C can be protective against cervical neoplasia
D have a consistently low failure rate
E should be used with a spermicide

(Answers overleaf)

2.138 A **False** In IVF the outcome increases with the number of
B **True** oocytes obtained. Ovulation induction is usually
C **False** perfomed using GnRH analogues (buserelin) and
D **True** gonadotrophins (pergonal). Under HFEA regulations
E **False** no more than three embryos can be replaced into
the uterus per cycle of treatment but the pregnancy
rate does increase with the number of embryos
replaced. Oocyte retrieval is usually performed
using a vaginal ultrasound under either a local or a
general anaesthetic. With superovulation it would
be desirable that all units were able to freeze any
extra embryos that were not replaced. Pregnancy
rates with IVF decrease markedly over the age of 40
and most units would suggest that women over the
age of 43 should use donor eggs.

2.139 A **True** Clomiphene citrate and tamoxifen are anti-
B **False** oestrogens used in high oestrogen states such as the
C **False** polycystic ovarian syndrome. Cyproterone acetate is
D **True** an anti-androgen used in treating virilism but not
E **True** ovulatory failure. Gonadotrophins may be used in
cases of pituitary failure or hypothalamic
amenorrhoea. Progesterone does not induce
ovulation.

2.140 A **True** Depo-Provera is an extremely effective (failure rate
B **True** less than 0.5 per 100 women years), reversible and
C **False** relatively safe method of contraception. In common
D **True** with all progestogens it can be used without an
E **False** upper age limit, in smokers, and when oestrogen is
contraindicated. Caution is advisable in women at
high risk of arterial disease. The main side effect is
breakthrough bleeding. Amenorrhoea occurs in 30%
of women after one year. It does not affect breast
feeding but there can be a delay in return to fertility
of up to 18 months.

2.141 A **False** Condoms are currently not available free from
B **False** general practitioners although they are available
C **True** from Health Authority Family Planning Clinics. The
D **False** failure rate can be very low but only if used
E **True** carefully and consistently. The condom should be
applied before any genital contact whatsoever and
spermicides should be used to enhance
effectiveness. They can be protective against
cervical neoplasia and sexually transmitted diseases.

2.142 Emergency contraception
- A is contraception used after intercourse but prior to implantation
- B when using oestrogens must be taken within 72 hours of intercourse
- C when using oestrogens, rarely has side effects
- D when using the IUCD must be inserted the 'morning after'
- E established contraindications to the oral contraceptive pill and the intrauterine contraceptive device still apply

2.143 During normal sexual intercourse
- A vaginal lubrication occurs from the cervical and vulval glands
- B uterine size increases
- C the orgasmic platform of the upper third of the vagina occurs
- D a sex flush appears around the perineum
- E the resolution phase preceeds orgasm

2.144 Progestogen only pills work as contraceptives by
- A suppressing ovulation
- B inducing cervical mucus hostility
- C producing endometrial hyperplasia
- D altering tubal motility
- E acting as a spermicide

2.145 Intrauterine contraceptive devices
- A prevent fertilisation
- B are teratogenic
- C need removing and replacing every two years
- D are contraindicated if there is a previous caesarean section scar
- E predispose to pelvic infection

2.146 Concerning natural family planning around the time of ovulation
- A cervical mucus is slippery with an elastic quality
- B basal body temperature may rise initially then show a prolonged drop
- C a woman may experience lower abdominal pain
- D luteinising hormone can be detected in the urine
- E the cervical mucus is impenetrable and hostile to sperm

(Answers overleaf)

2.142 A **True**   Hormonal emergency contraception consists of
     B **True**   200 µg of ethanyl oestradiol and 100 µg of
     C **False**   levonorgestrel given within 72 hours of intercourse.
     D **False**   The dose must be repeated 12 hours later. Nausea,
     E **False**   vomiting and mastalgia are common. Failure rate is
1–4%. The emergency IUCD may be fitted up to five
days after unprotected intercourse and fails in less
than 1% of cases. The emergency pill is
contraindicated when absolute contraindications to
oestrogen are present. It can, however, be used
with a past history of breast disease and arterial
disease. Discovery of an established pregnancy
provides the only absolute contraindication to
fitting an emergency IUCD provided the IUCD is
removed after the next period.

2.143 A **False**   The vaginal lubrication occurs as a transudation
     B **True**   through vaginal epithelium. The uterine size
     C **False**   increases. The upper third of the vagina balloons,
     D **False**   the lower third forms the orgasmic platform. 'Sex
     E **False**   flush' is a generalised skin hyperaemia and
resolution follows orgasm.

2.144 A **False**   Progestogen only pills rely for their contraceptive
     B **True**   action on inducing cervical mucus hostility
     C **False**   interfering with ovarian hormonal function without
     D **True**   necessarily suppressing ovulation, inducing
     E **False**   premature secretory changes in the endometrium
to prevent implantation and altering tubal motility.

2.145 A **False**   IUCDs act mainly by preventing implantation of the
     B **False**   fertilised ovum. There is no evidence of increased
     C **False**   risk of fetal abnormalities if the device fails,
     D **False**   although should the device remain in situ there is a
     E **True**   higher risk of miscarriage and pre-term delivery.
Inert IUCDs need not be replaced. Copper IUCDs
are licensed for 3–5 years although evidence is
increasingly suggesting use can be for up to seven
years.

2.146 A **True**   Natural family planning involves using the
     B **False**   physiological changes around the time of ovulation
     C **True**   to predict the period of increased fertility. At this
     D **True**   time the cervical mucus is slippery with an elastic
     E **False**   quality (spinbarkeit). It aids sperm motility. Basal
body temperature shows a drop, followed by a
prolonged rise. Some women may experience
ovulation pain (mittelschmerz). Home urine testing
kits are available over the counter in chemists to
detect the LH surge that accompanies ovulation.

2.147 A diaphragm or vaginal cap
A must be inserted six hours prior to intercourse
B should be fitted by a trained health professional
C protects against sexually transmitted disease
D is best used in conjunction with spermicides
E is as effective as hormonal contraception

2.148 Progestogen only oral contraceptive preparations
A are contraindicated in smokers over the age of 40
B are a suitable method of contraception for breast feeding women
C are as reliable as the combined oral contraceptive pill in preventing pregnancy
D are more reliable as the patient's age increases
E need to be taken at the same time each day

2.149 Vaginal secretions
A the pH becomes more alkaline prior to menstruation
B help to prevent pelvic inflammatory disease
C become more acidic in pregnancy
D come partly from secretions of the cervical glands
E are mainly secreted by vaginal glands

2.150 The following may reduce the effect of the combined oral contraceptive pill
A a pill taken six hours late
B penicillin
C anti-convulsant medication
D diarrhoea
E vaginal thrush

2.151 A 39-year-old smoker asks for contraceptive advice
A the combined oral contraceptive pill is contraindicated
B sterilisation is the only acceptable possibility
C an intrauterine contraceptive device should not be fitted
D a progesterone only contraceptive pill might be suitable
E barrier methods should be considered

(Answers overleaf)

2.147   A   **False**   A diaphragm or vaginal cap should be fitted by a
        B   **True**   trained professional who ensures that the woman is
        C   **True**   capable of fitting it correctly. It can be inserted
        D   **True**   immediately prior to intercourse but should remain
        E   **False**   in position for six hours afterwards. The device acts
                        as a barrier to sexually transmitted disease and in
                        addition the spermicide can kill pathogens. It is less
                        effective than hormonal contraception.

2.148   A   **False**   Progestogen only contraceptive preparations may
        B   **True**   be used by women of any age for whom oestrogen
        C   **False**   is contraindicated. Thus it may be a suitable
        D   **True**   method for smokers at any age and women with
        E   **True**   hypertension, diabetes or a history of
                        cardiovascular disease. It is also valuable during
                        lactation. Its main disadvantages are menstrual
                        irregularities and the need to take it at the same
                        time each day (within three hours). Its failure rate
                        decreases with age.

2.149   A   **True**   Vaginal fluid is a transudate through the vaginal
        B   **True**   epithelium along with desquamated cells, some
        C   **False**   polymorphs and bacterial flora and therefore not a
        D   **True**   secretion of vaginal glands. The acidity of the vagina
        E   **False**   provides a hostile environment for most bacteria and
                        therefore helps to prevent pelvic inflammatory
                        disease. The acid pH is maintained by the action of
                        Döderlein's bacilli on vaginal epithelial glycogen. The
                        secretions are less acidic prior to puberty,
                        postmenopausally and prior to and during
                        menstruation. Some secretions come from cervical
                        mucus as well as secretions from Skene's and
                        Bartholin's glands.

2.150   A   **False**   The absorption of combined oral contraceptive pills
        B   **True**   may be reduced with diarrhoea and short courses of
        C   **True**   broad spectrum antibiotics (by altering bowel flora).
        D   **True**   Any drug that induces liver enzymes, e.g. anti-
        E   **False**   convulsants, may reduce the efficacy of combined
                        oral contraceptives. Pill taking can be delayed by up
                        to 12 hours without loss of contraception.

2.151   A   **True**   After 35 years of age a smoker is in a high risk
        B   **False**   group for oestrogen induced hypertension and
        C   **False**   thrombosis. Progestogen only contraception,
        D   **True**   intrauterine devices and barrier methods are all
        E   **True**   suitable although they all have their failure rates.
                        Sterilisation may be the best alternative but the
                        patient should never be put under pressure to have
                        it performed.

2.152 The following are contraindications to using combined oral contraceptives
    A sickle-cell disease
    B porphyria
    C previous CIN III
    D depression
    E pulmonary embolus

2.153 Oral contraceptives containing oestrogens and progestogens
    A act by preventing ovulation
    B can cause hypertension
    C can cause venous thrombosis
    D usually cause amenorrhoea
    E reduce the viscosity of cervical mucus

2.154 Combined oral contraceptives are associated with
    A polymenorrhoea
    B menorrhagia
    C dysmenorrhoea
    D intermenstrual bleeding
    E ovarian cysts

2.155 Vasectomy
    A can be perfomed as an out-patient procedure
    B leads to immediate sterility
    C commonly causes impotence
    D involves ligation and division of the spermatic cord
    E can usually be successfully reversed 10 years after the original vasectomy

(Answers overleaf)

2.152 A **True**   Sickle-cell crises and attacks of porphyria may be
     B **True**   precipitated by oral contraceptives and they are
     C **False** best avoided in these patients. Because of the
     D **False** increased risk of thrombo-embolism in patients
     E **True**   taking these contraceptives they should be avoided
in those with a history of thrombosis or pulmonary
embolism. An association between CIN lesions and
oral contraceptives has been suggested but never
clearly demonstrated; the risk is likely to be very
low and effective. Contraception is often very
important in this group. There is no evidence that
oral contraceptives aggravate pre-existing
depression.

2.153 A **True**   Combined oral contraceptives usually prevent
     B **True**   ovulation and increase the viscosity of the cervical
     C **True**   mucus, making it relatively impenetrable to sperm.
     D **False** Mild, reversible hypertension is caused in between
     E **False** 1 and 5% of patients. Amenorrhoea is uncommon
and frequently not related to the contraceptives.
Venous thrombosis occurs more commonly in these
patients, particularly with pills containing higher
doses of oestrogens and in smokers.

2.154 A **False** Oral contraceptives contain oestrogens and
     B **False** progestogens cause regular, rather scanty
     C **False** withdrawal bleeds. Dysmenorrhoea is associated
     D **True**   with ovulatory cycles and oral contraceptives
     E **False** frequently relieve the symptom. The ovaries are
usually rather quiescent and certainly not cystic.
There may be breakthrough bleeding in the cycle
presenting as intermenstrual bleeding.

2.155 A **True**   Vasectomies are frequently performed as an
     B **False** out-patient procedure under local anaesthetic. The
     C **False** vas deferens is ligated and divided; if the spermatic
     D **False** cord were to be divided this would cut the blood
     E **False** supply to the testis. The sperm count declines
gradually and it may take several months for
infertility to be total, depending upon the frequency
of ejaculation. If vasectomy caused impotence it
would scarcely be so popular. After 10 years the
chances of successful reversal become very low
and levels of sperm antibodies are very high.

2.156 Under the 1991 revision of the 1967 Abortion Act

    A abortion can be performed at any gestation to save the life of the pregnant mother

    B abortion can be performed at 27 weeks because of the risk of severe psychiatric illness in the mother

    C abortion can be performed following rubella infection in the first trimester

    D the GP and hospital practitioner are required to certify the need for abortion

    E a patient may not have more than two abortions

2.157 Medical termination of pregnancy

    A involves the use of mifepristone alone

    B requires a surgical evacuation of the uterus in 5–10% of cases

    C is much cheaper than surgical termination of pregnancy

    D may occur at home

    E is painless

(Answers overleaf)

2.156 A **True**   The Act requires two registered medical
     B **False**   practitioners to sign the forms certifying that an
     C **True**   abortion is necessary. This is often the GP and
     D **False**   hospital practitioner but may be two hospital
     E **False**   practitioners. An abortion can be performed to
prevent grave permanent injury to the physical or
mental health of the woman or to save the life of
the pregnant woman at any gestation. An abortion
can be performed prior to 24 weeks if the
continuation of the pregnancy would involve risk
greater than if the pregnancy were terminated, of
injury to the physical or mental health of the
pregnant woman or to the physical or mental
health of any existing children of the family of the
pregnant woman. An abortion can be performed at
any gestation if there is a substantial risk that if the
child were born it would suffer from such physical
or mental abnormalities as to be seriously
handicapped. There is no stipulation on the number
of abortions that a lady may have.

2.157 A **False**   Medical termination of pregnancy involves full
     B **True**   counselling of the patient. The normal criteria under
     C **False**   the terms of the Abortion Act need to be fulfilled.
     D **False**   Mifepristone 600 mg is then given to the lady. She is
     E **False**   readmitted 36–48 hours later and a pessary
containing Gemeprost 1 mg is inserted into the
vagina. 90% of women will abort within six hours. The
abortion that follows mifepristone and Gemeprost
resembles a spontaneous miscarriage and will be
complete, requiring no surgical intervention, in 95%
of cases. Narcotic analgesics are needed in one-third
of women. Medical abortion can be performed up to
and including the ninth week of amenorrhoea. The
abortion must occur on NHS or licensed premises.
There seems to be little in terms of cost between
medical terminations and surgical terminations of
pregnancy but many women would prefer the former.

2.158 Surgical termination of pregnancy
A should be completely replaced by medical termination of pregnancy
B requires a re-evacuation of the uterus in 5–10% of cases
C is usually performed by suction evacuation of the uterus
D is best performed at 12–13 weeks of gestation
E post-evacuation pelvic inflammatory disease can be decreased if chlamydia is isolated and treated prior to the procedure

PROBLEMS OF EARLY PREGNANCY

2.159 First trimester spontaneous abortions are due to
A trisomies
B triploidies
C placental abruption
D pregnancy induced hypertension
E rubella infection

2.160 In case of threatened abortion
A pain is absent
B bleeding is always slight
C the cervical os is closed
D the pregnancy continues in most cases
E admission to hospital is necessary

2.161 A patient with a missed abortion
A usually presents complaining of a diminution in fetal movements
B has a significant risk of uterine haemorrhage due to coagulopathy
C will develop a septic abortion if the uterus is not emptied within seven days
D usually has a uterus smaller than would be expected from her dates
E often presents with a brown vaginal discharge

(Answers overleaf)

2.158 A **False**   Medical termination cannot be performed after nine
      B **True**   weeks of gestation and there will always be a place
      C **True**   for both procedures. The re-evacuation rate is 5–10%
      D **False**   which is similar to the evacuation rate following a
      E **True**   medical termination of pregnancy. The uterus is
                     usually emptied by suction evacuation of the uterus
                     following cervical dilatation. It is best performed
                     between seven and 11 weeks and the complication
                     rate increases after this time. Women should have an
                     endocervical swab taken for chlamydia prior to a
                     suction termination of pregnancy and if the organism
                     is isolated and treated the incidence of PID is
                     decreased.

PROBLEMS OF EARLY PREGNANCY

2.159 A **True**   30% of first trimester spontaneous abortions are
      B **True**   due to trisomies and in 10% of cases there is
      C **False**   polyploidy, mostly triploidy. Rubella infection, in
      D **False**   addition to causing congenital abnormalities, is well
      E **True**   known for causing spontaneous abortion. Placental
                     abruption occurs much later in pregnancy as does
                     pregnancy induced hypertension.

2.160 A **False**   Although pain and heavy bleeding are always
      B **False**   worrying features, neither are diagnostic of
      C **True**   inevitable abortion. Approximately 70% of patients
      D **True**   will go on to have normal pregnancies after a
      E **False**   threatened abortion. The diagnosis rests on the
                     presence of a live fetus and the cervical os being
                     closed. Most cases can be, and are, managed at
                     home.

2.161 A **False**   Patients with missed abortions usually present with
      B **False**   a small for dates uterus, with or without vaginal
      C **False**   bleeding, commonly of old blood, usually before 16
      D **True**   weeks gestation. Infection will only be introduced at
      E **True**   curettage, not before. Hypofibrinogenaemia can
                     develop if treatment is delayed for several weeks,
                     but is very uncommon.

2.162 Incomplete abortion

A is treated by suction curettage
B inevitably leads to the development of pelvic infection unless treated with antibiotics
C is common before seven weeks gestation
D is usually diagnosed by ultrasound scan
E is commonest in the first trimester of pregnancy

2.163 Recurrent first trimester abortion is caused by

A cervical incompetence
B uncontrolled diabetes mellitus
C uterine structural abnormalities
D uterine fibroids
E a balanced translocation in one parent

2.164 Organisms involved in septic abortions often include

A *E. coli*
B haemolytic streptococci
C *Clostridium perfringens*
D *Mycobacterium tuberculosis*
E *N. gonorrhoeae*

2.165 The treatment of septic abortion may include

A emptying the uterus
B intravenous administration of antibiotics
C corticosteroids
D control of metabolic alkalosis
E blood transfusion

2.166 Lower abdominal pain in the first 10 weeks of pregnancy may be due to

A acute appendicitis
B an ectopic pregnancy
C an impacted retroverted uterus
D acute salpingitis
E spontaneous abortion

2.167 A patient with an impacted retroverted uterus in pregnancy

A presents with urinary retention
B is treated best by termination of pregnancy
C usually has co-existing uterine fibroids
D can be reassured as the condition will usually resolve with adequate treatment
E should be admitted to hospital

(Answers overleaf)

2.162 A **True**   Incomplete abortion occurs most commonly in the
       B **False** first trimester, but before eight weeks most cases of
       C **False** abortion are complete and do not present to the
       D **False** hospital. Diagnosis is clinical (bleeding, open
       E **True**   cervical os) and ultrasound is not necessary. Pelvic
                     infection may occur, but should be uncommon.

2.163 A **False** Cervical incompetence and uterine structural
       B **True**   abnormalities more commonly cause abortion in
       C **False** the second trimester or alternatively cause
       D **True**   premature labour. Balanced translocations in a
       E **True**   parent may lead to unbalanced translocations in the
                     fetus and subsequent abortion. Uterine fibroids
                     may cause difficulties with implantation.

2.164 A **True**   Septic abortion occurs because of introduction of
       B **True**   infection into the uterus, usually during an attempt,
       C **True**   legal or otherwise, to procure abortion. If the uterus
       D **False** is not emptied the retained products are a good
       E **False** culture medium. Consequently, the organisms
                     involved are those most commonly found in the
                     area, often as commensals until introduced into the
                     uterus.

2.165 A **True**   Septic abortion is a serious condition that may be
       B **True**   life threatening. Treatment is with intravenous
       C **True**   antibiotics, followed by evacuation of retained
       D **False** products. If Gram-negative septicaemia has
       E **True**   developed, measures may need to be taken to
                     correct acidosis, correct coagulopathies and deal
                     with shock, including corticosteroids and blood
                     transfusion.

2.166 A **True**   Pain in early pregnancy may be due to
       B **True**   complications of pregnancy, abortion or ectopic, or
       C **False** coincidental problems such as acute appendicitis.
       D **False** Salpingitis is very uncommon in pregnancy. An
       E **True**   impacted, retroverted uterus presents at 13 to 14
                     weeks.

2.167 A **True**   Patients with impacted retroversion usually present
       B **False** with urinary retention at 13 to 14 weeks gestation.
       C **False** The patient must be admitted to hospital and the
       D **True**   bladder catheterised. Emptying the bladder leaves
       E **True**   more space for the uterus in the pelvis and the
                     condition will resolve in two or three days.
                     Traditionally the patient is nursed lying on her front
                     for most of the time, but it is not clear that this
                     makes any difference.

2.168 Bleeding in early pregnancy could be caused by
A an ectopic pregnancy
B hydatidiform mole
C carcinoma of the ovary
D invasive carcinoma of the cervix
E cervical intraepithelial neoplasia

2.169 Ectopic pregnancy
A occurs in 1 in 400 pregnancies in the United Kingdom
B is most commonly sited in the fallopian tube
C usually presents with shock and collapse
D is the commonest type of pregnancy when there is an intrauterine contraceptive device in place
E may occur in the cervical canal

2.170 The risk of developing ectopic pregnancy is increased in patients who have had
A pelvic infection
B tubal surgery for infertility
C sterilisation
D a previous ectopic pregnancy
E an intrauterine contraceptive device inserted during the previous three months

2.171 Signs and symptoms of ectopic pregnancy include
A heavy vaginal bleeding
B pyrexia
C tachycardia
D cervical excitation
E bilateral pelvic pain

2.172 When a patient collapses at home with a suspected ruptured ectopic pregnancy
A the obstetric flying squad should be called
B the attending doctor should perform a vaginal examination to confirm the diagnosis
C the patient should be transferred to hospital for resuscitation
D transfer to hospital and immediate laparotomy is indicated
E intravenous ergometrine should be given

(Answers overleaf)

2.168 A **True** Bleeding in early pregnancy may be due to
      B **True** abortion, ectopic pregnancy, trophoblastic disease
      C **False** or coincidental causes such as invasive cancer of
      D **True** the cervix. Cervical intraepithelial neoplasia is
      E **False** asymptomatic.

2.169 A **False** Ectopic pregnancy occurs in approximately 1 in 200
      B **True** pregnancies in the United Kingdom, although it is
      C **False** becoming more common. Most ectopics are in the
      D **False** fallopian tube although they can occur in the ovary,
      E **True** in the abdominal cavity or, rarely, in the cervical
                  canal. Most cases present subacutely with pain and
                  bleeding and presentation with collapse is unusual.
                  When a pregnant patient has an IUCD in place the
                  likelihood of ectopic pregnancy is increased, but
                  intrauterine pregnancy is still far more common.

2.170 A **True** Tubal damage causes ectopic pregnancy, whether
      B **True** caused by infection or surgery. Once present,
      C **False** aetiological factors will continue to make recurrent
      D **True** ectopic pregnancy more likely. Although when
      E **False** sterilised patients get pregnant they have a higher
                  incidence of ectopics, they become pregnant only
                  rarely. The increase in the ectopic rate that is
                  sometimes blamed on IUCDs is related to old or
                  chronic PID. It is unlikely to be seen in the short
                  term.

2.171 A **False** In ectopic pregnancies vaginal bleeding is usually
      B **False** relatively slight. Pyrexia is unusual although there
      C **True** is often a tachycardia. The patient may complain of
      D **True** unilateral pelvic pain initially but this soon becomes
      E **True** bilateral and there is marked cervical excitation on
                  vaginal examination.

2.172 A **True** Collapse with a ruptured ectopic at home is a major
      B **False** catastrophe and the patient should be resuscitated
      C **False** as far as possible at home by the flying squad, but
      D **True** this should not delay transfer to hospital for
      E **False** immediate laparotomy. Once in hospital
                  resuscitation and surgery go hand in hand, there is
                  no point in delaying surgery. Vaginal examination
                  at home may exacerbate the bleeding and is rarely
                  necessary. Ergometrine makes the uterus contract
                  and is useless for tubal bleeding.

2.173 In the investigation of a suspected ectopic pregnancy
A a vaginal ultrasound scan is useful
B serum beta HCG estimation is of value
C the patient will be anaemic
D laparoscopy is essential
E the diagnosis is usually obvious from the history

2.174 Hydatidiform mole presents
A as a coincidental finding on ultrasound scan
B with vaginal bleeding
C with pelvic pain
D as a small for dates uterus at booking
E as hypothyroidism

2.175 Partial hydatidiform mole
A may develop into complete mole
B is chromosomally 46XX
C may be accompanied by a fetus in utero
D is less common than complete mole
E will develop into choriocarcinoma in 5% of cases

2.176 Complete hydatidiform mole
A has a genetic complement entirely derived from the father
B is chromosomally 46XX
C does not co-exist with an embryo
D occurs in approximately 1 in 3500 pregnancies in the United Kingdom
E characteristically invades the myometrium

(Answers overleaf)

2.173 A **True**   Clinical diagnosis of an ectopic pregnancy may be
      B **True**   easy in some cases but in many it is notoriously
      C **False**   difficult. Whilst laparoscopy is essential if there is
      D **False**   any doubt, pregnancy test using serum beta HCG
      E **False**   estimation is almost invariably positive in ectopic
pregnancies and this, coupled with a vaginal
ultrasound scan showing an empty uterus, will
make ectopic pregnancy very likely as the
diagnosis. If the beta HCG is negative or the vaginal
ultrasound scan shows a pregnancy within the
uterus laparoscopy is unlikely to be necessary. In
many cases of subacute presentation the patient
may not be anaemic.

2.174 A **True**   Nowadays hydatidiform mole is frequently seen on
      B **True**   ultrasound scan. The commonest presentation,
      C **True**   however, is vaginal bleeding. It is associated with
      D **False**   theca-lutein cysts which may rupture or tort and
      E **False**   cause pain. The uterus is large for dates.
Occasionally HCG levels may be high enough to
increase thyroid function.

2.175 A **False**   Partial hydatidiform mole is an entity completely
      B **False**   separate from complete mole. Complete mole is
      C **True**   chromosomally 46XX whereas partial mole is
      D **True**   triploid. Partial moles are accompanied by a fetus in
      E **False**   utero although the fetus usually dies at an early
stage of the pregnancy. The condition is less
common than complete mole and there are no
recorded cases of development of choriocarcinoma
after partial mole, although in many centres these
patients are followed for a while in order to ensure
that there is no persistent trophoblastic disease.

2.176 A **True**   Complete hydatidiform mole has a genetic
      B **True**   complement which is probably derived from two
      C **True**   sperms entering an oocyte with no genetic material of
      D **False**   its own. Consequently, although the mole is
      E **False**   chromosomally 46XX (46XY moles do not generally
survive) all of these chromosomes have been derived
from the father. An embryo is not present. In the
United Kingdom hydatidiform mole occurs in
approximately 1 in 1500 pregnancies. If invasion of
the myometrium occurs this is known as an invasive
mole.

2.177 Choriocarcinoma

    A   is usually treated by hysterectomy
    B   has a very poor prognosis even with adequate treatment
    C   may present with haemoptysis
    D   metastasises to the vagina
    E   is an absolute contraindication to future pregnancy

2.178 Invasive mole

    A   usually follows hydatidiform mole
    B   may metastasise to the lungs
    C   is synonymous with choriocarcinoma
    D   may present with vaginal bleeding
    E   does not secrete HCG

(Answers overleaf)

2.177 A **False**   Treatment is with cytotoxic agents and the
      B **False**   prognosis is excellent. Metastases occur early and
      C **True**   the patient may present with a nodule in the vagina
      D **True**   or lung secondaries causing haemoptysis. Once
      E **False**   adequately treated the patient may become
      pregnant again, although many may choose not to.

2.178 A **True**   Invasive mole can be differentiated from
      B **True**   choriocarcinoma histologically. It almost always
      C **False**   follows hydatidiform mole (unlike choriocarcinoma)
      D **True**   and deposits may be seen in the lungs and pelvic
      E **False**   organs. Patients may have vaginal bleeding,
      amenorrhoea, infertility and abdominal pain. As
      with other forms of trophoblastic disease HCG is
      secreted.

3. Obstetrics

3.1 Preconceptual counselling
A should be reserved for 'high risk' patients
B should include a check on rubella immunity
C is best performed in the hospital antenatal clinic
D should include advice about smoking
E should include an HIV test

3.2 The hospital antenatal booking clinic visit should
A occur in the first trimester
B should include a general examination
C is important as a screening procedure
D should ensure that all women are taking oral iron supplementation
E should include a vaginal examination

3.3 The following routine investigations should be performed at the antenatal booking visit
A haemoglobin estimation
B HIV test
C HCG estimation
D syphilis serology
E ABO and Rhesus blood grouping

3.4 A 14 week ultrasound scan
A should be performed in all pregnancies
B usually takes about 30 minutes to perform
C is important to assess liquor volume
D allows gestational age to be calculated accurately by crown rump length
E involves placental localisation

(Answers overleaf)

3.1 A **False**   Preconception clinics allow women with medical
    B **True**   disorders to become pregnant in as healthy a
    C **False**   condition as possible, offer dietary advice,
    D **True**   encourage women to decrease smoking and alcohol
    E **False**   intake, advise about previous pregnancy
             complications and check rubella immunity.
             Preconceptual counselling is best performed by the
             GP in the majority of cases. An HIV test should only
             be performed on those patients with risk factors
             after permission from the patient.

3.2 A **False**   The hospital booking clinic visit is an important
    B **True**   screening procedure as an accurate history and
    C **True**   examination with appropriate investigations will
    D **False**   indicate women at risk of pregnancy complications.
    E **False**   It is usually arranged at 16 to 18 weeks, when the
             woman has passed the risk of early miscarriage
             and the visit can be combined with a detailed
             ultrasound scan. A vaginal examination is only
             necessary when there are clinical indications. Only
             women with proven iron deficiency anaemia or
             those at significant risk of developing this require
             oral iron supplementation.

3.3 A **True**   At the booking visit a haemoglobin estimation and
    B **False**   blood grouping should be checked on all patients. If
    C **False**   the patient is Rhesus negative then antibody titres
    D **True**   should be checked. Serological testing should be
    E **True**   performed for syphilis and for rubella but an HIV
             test and HCG estimation are not performed
             routinely.

3.4 A **False**   A level 1 scan should be performed in all women in
    B **False**   pregnancy unless a level 2 scan is being performed
    C **False**   at 18 weeks. It usually takes about 10 minutes to
    D **False**   perform and it is a good screening procedure for
    E **True**   fetal abnormality, multiple pregnancy and fetal
             viability. Changes in liquor volume usually occur
             after the first trimester. After the first trimester
             measurement of crown rump length relates less
             well to dates because of flexion of the fetus and it
             is usual to measure the biparietal diameter and
             femur length to obtain an accurate gestation.
             Placental localisation at this stage can help but
             these women should be re-scanned later in
             pregnancy.

3.5   Vomiting in early pregnancy
   A   occurs more frequently with trophoblastic disease
   B   increases with gravidity
   C   is associated with multiple pregnancy
   D   usually settles by the tenth week of pregnancy
   E   increases with maternal age

3.6   Alphafetoprotein concentration increases in
   A   maternal serum in the second trimester
   B   the amniotic fluid in the second trimester
   C   amniotic fluid in the presence of all neural tube defects
   D   maternal serum in multiple pregnancy
   E   amniotic fluid in cases of gastroschisis

3.7   At 14 weeks gestation a uterus may feel large for dates because of
   A   wrong dates
   B   uterine fibroids
   C   polyhydramnios
   D   multiple pregnancy
   E   diabetes mellitus

3.8   Down syndrome
   A   is the commonest chromosomal abnormality
   B   can be diagnosed by the 'triple blood test' at 16 weeks
   C   most children with Down syndrome are born to women over 35 years of age
   D   is always due to trisomy 21
   E   is a common cause of first trimester miscarriage

3.9   An increased risk of a baby being born with Down syndrome is associated with
   A   increasing paternal age
   B   increasing maternal age
   C   a reduced maternal serum alphafetoprotein at 16 weeks gestation
   D   a reduced serum HCG at 16 weeks gestation
   E   a previous baby affected with Down syndrome

(Answers overleaf)

3.5 A **True**   Vomiting in pregnancy usually occurs maximally
     B **False** between the 8th and 14th week of gestation. It is
     C **True**   commonest in first pregnancies and is unrelated to
     D **False** maternal age. It is associated with multiple
     E **False** pregnancy and trophoblastic disease.

3.6 A **True**   Maternal serum alphafetoprotein concentrations
     B **False** increase with gestation. They are abnormally raised
     C **False** in multiple pregnancies and with various fetal
     D **True**   abnormalities. Amniotic fluid alphafetoprotein levels
     E **True**   reach a peak at 13 to 14 weeks and then fall with
                   gestation. They are pathologically increased by
                   open neural tube defects and some other
                   abnormalities including exomphalos and
                   gastroschisis.

3.7 A **True**   When the uterus feels large at 14 weeks it is usually
     B **True**   due to wrong dates, but can be caused by pelvic
     C **False** masses, a full bladder, fibroids or ovarian cysts.
     D **True**   Multiple pregnancies begin to be detectable at this
     E **False** stage but the enlargement caused by
                   polyhydramnios or diabetes occurs at a later stage
                   of gestation.

3.8 A **True**   Down syndrome is the commonest chromosomal
     B **False** abnormality and is associated with first trimester
     C **False** miscarriage. In 95% of cases it is due to trisomy 21,
     D **False** although translocations make up 4% and mosaicism
     E **True**   1% of children born with this condition. Three
                   quarters of children with Down syndrome are born
                   to mothers under the age of 35 years. The
                   incidence increases after the age of 35 years. The
                   triple blood test can give a relative risk of Down
                   syndrome but is not a diagnostic test. A karyotype,
                   performed following CVS or amniocentesis, is the
                   standard diagnostic test.

3.9 A **False** The risk of a baby having Down syndrome is
     B **True**   increased with maternal age. A previously affected
     C **True**   child gives a risk of recurrence due to trisomy 21 of
     D **False** 1 in a 100 but a risk of about 1 in 10 if it is due to a
     E **True**   balanced translocation in the mother. A raised
                   serum HCG and a reduced serum alphafetoprotein
                   at 16 weeks are used in conjunction with maternal
                   age and gestation to calculate the relative risk of
                   Down syndrome in the 'double test'. The 'triple test'
                   includes a serum oestriol estimation.

3.10 Amniocentesis

    A   must be performed on all women over 37 years of age
    B   is usually performed at 16–18 weeks of gestation
    C   carries a 5% risk of causing a miscarriage
    D   should not be followed by an injection of anti-D in Rhesus negative women
    E   is best performed transplacentally

3.11 The following disorders can be diagnosed antenatally by amniocentesis

    A   Duchenne muscular dystrophy
    B   Turner's syndrome
    C   closed neural tube defects
    D   glucose-6-phosphate dehydrogenase deficiency
    E   tracheo-oesophageal fistula

3.12 Chorionic villus sampling

    A   is usually performed transabdominally
    B   is best performed before 10 weeks of gestation
    C   usually reveals a karyotype within 24 hours
    D   carries a procedure related miscarriage rate of 1%
    E   involves a suction aspiration of 5–10 mg of chorionic villi

3.13 An 18 week detailed (level 2) ultrasound scan should

    A   be able to diagnose Potter's syndrome
    B   detect a closed spina bifida
    C   be able to determine fetal sex
    D   ideally be performed on all antenatal patients
    E   detect a diaphragmatic hernia

(Answers overleaf)

3.10 A **False** Amniocentesis is usually carried out between 16–18
    B **True** weeks of gestation. It should be performed under
    C **False** ultrasound control and the placenta should be
    D **False** avoided if possible. The procedure carries a risk of
    E **False** miscarriage over the background rate of about 1%.
Although it is generally offered to women over 35
years of age, it is the patient's choice as to whether
they wish this to be performed. There is a risk of
isoimmunisation in Rhesus negative women and a
Kleihauer should be performed 20 minutes after the
procedure. Anti-D immunoglobulin should be given
to all Rhesus negative women.

3.11 A **False** A fetal karyotype will demonstrate Turner's
    B **True** syndrome and other chromosomal abnormalities as
    C **False** well as the sex of the fetus. It will only indicate the
    D **True** at risk group (male) for muscular dystrophy.
    E **False** Alphafetoprotein measurement will diagnose open
neural tube defects. In G6PD deficiency lack of the
enzyme can be demonstrated. Tracheo-oesophageal
fistula may cause polyhydramnios, but no changes
on amniocentesis.

3.12 A **False** At the present time the majority of centres still use
    B **False** a transcervical approach for CVS. There is,
    C **True** however, an increasing use of the transabdominal
    D **False** approach. This is because of the theoretical
    E **True** advantage of reducing infection, as well as better
acceptance by patients and doctors and the ability
to use the procedure throughout pregnancy. There
have been several severe limb abnormalities
reported in babies whose mothers have undergone
early CVS and so the procedure is now not usually
performed before 10 weeks gestation. A direct
preparation, or short term culture, will reveal
karyotype results in 12 to 24 hours. These results
are always checked with a long term culture, the
result of which usually takes about a week. The
procedure related miscarriage rate for CVS is about
3.5%.

3.13 A **True** An 18 week level 2 detailed scan should ideally be
    B **True** performed in all women in pregnancy and usually
    C **True** takes about 30 minutes to perform. About 1 in 5
    D **True** need to be repeated one or two weeks later
    E **True** because of the attitude of the fetus. The scanner
should be able to detect cranio-spinal,
gastrointestinal, renal, urinary tract and cardiac
abnormalities as well as limb deformities.

3.14 A 38-year-old woman in her first pregnancy

A   should always be delivered in hospital
B   should be offered amniocentesis
C   would frequently have significant anaemia
D   should be delivered by caesarean section
E   is more likely than average to develop hypertension

3.15 At each routine hospital antenatal visit in the third trimester the following should be assessed

A   patient awareness of fetal movement
B   the biparietal diameter of the fetus
C   the fundal height
D   the presentation of the fetus
E   haemoglobin estimation

3.16 Multiple pregnancy

A   occurs in approximately 1 in 80 pregnancies
B   is commoner in older women
C   is usually monozygotic following IVF
D   is frequently complicated by premature labour
E   is associated with an increased risk of primary postpartum haemorrhage

3.17 A diagnosis of twin pregnancy may confidently be made

A   after ultrasound examination
B   on finding two fetal heads at clinical examination
C   when the uterus is found to be large for dates
D   after X-ray of the abdomen
E   on hearing the fetal heart at two separate sites on the maternal abdomen

3.18 Multiple pregnancies predispose to

A   placenta praevia
B   diabetes mellitus
C   acute pyelonephritis
D   placental insufficiency
E   malpresentation

3.19 Erect lateral X-ray pelvimetry

A   is necessary for the diagnosis of cephalo-pelvic disproportion
B   will reveal the bispinous diameter
C   is usually performed between 28 and 32 weeks
D   is rarely of value in an uncomplicated pregnancy when the fetus presents by the head
E   may be necessary when the patient has had a previous caesarean section

(Answers overleaf)

3.14 A **True**   The risks of pregnancy, particularly of developing
      B **True**   hypertension, increase with age. Amniocentesis is
      C **False** offered because of the increasing risk of
      D **False** chromosomal disorders at this age (1.4%). Most of
      E **True**   these pregnancies, however, are entirely normal.

3.15 A **True**   An assessment should be made of the fundal
      B **False** height, the presentation and lie of the fetus and the
      C **True**   presence of the fetal heartbeat. The biparietal
      D **True**   diameter should be measured by ultrasound scan if
      E **False** the fundal height is large or small for the expected
                    gestation. A haemoglobin estimation should be
                    performed monthly, but not at every antenatal visit.

3.16 A **True**   Twins occur in approximately 1 in 80 pregnancies.
      B **True**   Premature labour is common and is a major cause
      C **False** of perinatal mortality in twins. The size of the
      D **True**   placental bed and over-distention of the uterus
      E **True**   combine to cause an increased risk of post partum
                    haemorrhage. Spontaneous twins are commoner in
                    older women and are usually dizygotic following IVF.

3.17 A **True**   To diagnose twins clinically at least three fetal poles
      B **False** must be felt. The uterus may be large for dates for
      C **False** a variety of reasons. To be sure of hearing two fetal
      D **True**   hearts they must be heard simultaneously by two
      E **False** people and have different rates. Ultrasound or
                    X-ray reliably diagnoses twins.

3.18 A **True**   The greater placental area makes placenta praevia
      B **False** more likely. Acute pyelonephritis, placental
      C **True**   insufficiency, hypertension, polyhydramnios,
      D **True**   malpresentations and prematurity are all more
      E **True**   common. There is no association between twins
                    and diabetes.

3.19 A **False** Cephalo-pelvic disproportion is a diagnosis which
      B **False** can be made following a trial of labour with good
      C **False** uterine contractions. Lateral X-ray pelvimetry is
      D **True**   therefore not necessary to make this diagnosis. An
      E **True**   AP X-ray will reveal the bispinous diameter and not
                    a lateral X-ray. Unless the pelvis is extremely small,
                    in a cephalic presentation a trial of labour will be
                    performed and there is little correlation between
                    cephalo-pelvic disproportion on X-ray and failed
                    vaginal delivery. A scarred uterus or breech
                    presentation is often an indication for X-ray
                    pelvimetry to ensure that there is no question of 'a
                    tight fit'. There is really no indication to perform
                    pelvimetry prior to 36 weeks of gestation.

3.20 Oligohydramnios is associated with
A   multiple pregnancy
B   diabetes mellitus
C   postmaturity
D   renal agenesis
E   oesophageal atresia

3.21 Polyhydramnios in the third trimester is associated with
A   diabetes mellitus
B   intrauterine growth retardation
C   Rhesus disease
D   amniocentesis at 16 weeks gestation
E   fetal neural tube defect

3.22 The following factors are associated with an increased risk of adverse outcome to the baby and/or the mother
A   girls under 18 years of age
B   an unmarried mother
C   grandmultiparity
D   previous large baby
E   a height of 1.6 metres or more

3.23 The following factors affect birthweight
A   fetal sex
B   the altitude at which the mother lives
C   ethnic origin
D   dieting in pregnancy
E   multiple pregnancy

3.24 The following may adversely affect pregnancy outcome
A   smoking
B   maternal alcohol consumption of 3 units daily
C   consumption of paté
D   genital herpes
E   sexual intercourse in the third trimester

3.25 Spontaneous premature labour is associated with
A   low socio-economic class
B   multiple pregnancy
C   placenta praevia
D   congenital uterine abnormalities
E   cervical incompetence

(Answers overleaf)

3.20 A **False** Oligohydramnios is associated with some fetal
     B **False** abnormalities, including Potter's syndrome (renal
     C **True**   agenesis), intrauterine growth retardation and post-
     D **True**   maturity. Polyhydramnios is associated with twins,
     E **False** oesophageal atresia and diabetes.

3.21 A **True**   Polyhydramnios is associated with Rhesus disease,
     B **False** diabetes, twins and some fetal abnormalities
     C **True**   including anencephaly. Intrauterine growth
     D **False** retardation is associated with oligohydramnios.
     E **True**   Early amniocentesis is said to be associated with
                    oligohydramnios in a few cases because of
                    continued leakage of liquor.

3.22 A **True**   Girls under the age of 18 years, unmarried women,
     B **True**   women on their fifth or subsequent delivery or who
     C **True**   previously had an infant larger than 4 kg have an
     D **True**   increased perinatal mortality rate. Women who are
     E **False** below 1.52 metres in height have an increased
                    perinatal mortality rate but a height of 1.6 metres is
                    not associated with an adverse outcome.

3.23 A **True**   Gestation and parity affect birthweight and boys
     B **True**   matched for both weigh more than girls. Children
     C **True**   born to mothers who live at high altitudes or of
     D **False** certain ethnic origins, e.g. Hindu women, are
     E **True**   smaller. Dieting, assuming that it is not a starvation
                    diet, does not affect birthweight. Babies from a
                    multiple pregnancy are smaller than a singleton
                    matched for other variables.

3.24 A **True**   Smoking in pregnancy affects birthweight and
     B **True**   perinatal mortality. Alcohol consumption greater
     C **True**   than 2 units daily is associated with decreased
     D **True**   birthweight whilst high consumption greater than 6
     E **False** units daily can lead to the fetal alcohol syndrome.
                    Paté not only contains liver (which has high levels
                    of vitamin A) but may also harbour listeria. Active
                    genital herpes in labour is an indication for
                    caesarean section. In cases of placenta praevia,
                    APH and premature rupture of membranes sexual
                    intercourse in the third trimester should be avoided,
                    but otherwise it has no deleterious effect on
                    pregnancy outcome.

3.25 A **True**   Spontaneous premature labour can be caused by
     B **True**   poor social factors, an incompetent cervix, uterine
     C **False** abnormalities, twins, polyhydramnios, maternal
     D **True**   pyrexia, some fetal abnormalities and intrauterine
     E **True**   fetal death.

3.26 Premature labour
A   is defined as any labour commencing before 37 completed weeks of pregnancy
B   is the leading cause of perinatal mortality in the UK
C   occurs in approximately 6% of all pregnancies
D   should always be suppressed
E   if it occurs before 32 weeks of pregnancy, babies are best delivered by caesarean section

3.27 Suppression of premature labour with a beta-sympathomimetic agent, e.g. ritodrine
A   may lead to maternal glycosuria
B   should not be used if the cervix is more than 2 cm dilated
C   has been shown to increase the length of pregnancy by about one week
D   would not usually be performed after 34 weeks
E   should not be performed with spontaneous rupture of the membranes

(Answers overleaf)

3.26 A **True** Preterm labour is defined as labour commencing
     B **True** before 37 completed weeks of gestation. It is the
     C **True** leading cause of perinatal mortality in the UK and
     D **False** occurs in 6–10% of all pregnancies. If the woman is
     E **False** over 34 weeks gestation or if the cervix is greater
              than 5 cm dilated, if there is premature rupture of
              membranes, if there has been bleeding or if the
              fetus is dead no attempt should be made to
              suppress the labour. Suppression of labour is
              controversial but may prolong the pregnancy for
              about 24 hours perhaps allowing maternal steroids
              to decrease the chance of respiratory distress
              syndrome in the infant. If babies present by the
              breech there is evidence that between 28 and 32
              weeks they are better off delivered by caesarean
              section, but if they present by the vertex then
              standard criteria should be used for caesarean
              section.

3.27 A **True** Suppression of labour after 34 weeks is generally
     B **False** not performed unless an in utero transfer is being
     C **False** considered to another hospital. Beta-
     D **True** sympathomimetic agents should not be used if
     E **True** there is an abnormal CTG, ruptured membranes, an
              antepartum haemorrhage, the cervix is greater than
              5 cm dilated or if there is significant cardiac disease
              or diabetes mellitus. The side effects in the mother
              are of tachycardia, tremor and glycosuria. The
              evidence is that suppression of labour, with beta-
              sympathomimetic agents, prolongs pregnancy by
              about 24 hours. There is considerable debate as to
              whether this is worthwhile in view of the side
              effects. However, it may well allow time for steroids
              to be administered to the mother and to allow
              some fetal lung maturation.

3.28 **The following drugs will suppress uterine contractions**
  A   salbutamol
  B   indomethacin
  C   dexamethasone
  D   alcohol
  E   pethidine

3.29 **Antepartum haemorrhage**
  A   occurs in 1% of pregnancies
  B   may occur from the 24th week of pregnancy
  C   may occur during the second stage of labour
  D   almost always leads to loss of maternal rather than fetal loss of blood
  E   may be caused by carcinoma of the cervix

3.30 **Placental abruption**
  A   is common in the first trimester of pregnancy
  B   is called 'accidental' because of its association with trauma
  C   is associated with postpartum haemorrhage
  D   can be treated with beta-adrenergic drugs
  E   may not present as vaginal bleeding

3.31 **The patient with a severe placental abruption and a dead fetus should be**
  A   given a liberal blood transfusion
  B   given analgesics
  C   put to bed to await the spontaneous onset of labour
  D   have her forewaters ruptured
  E   be given an intravenous Syntocinon infusion

(Answers overleaf)

3.28 A **True**   Beta-sympathomimetic agents, e.g. salbutamol and
      B **True**   ritodrine, are used to suppress uterine contractions.
      C **False** They should not be used if the cervix is greater
      D **True**   than 5 cm dilated, if there is spontaneous rupture of
      E **False** the membranes or if the woman has had an
                    antepartum haemorrhage. They must be used with
                    caution in women with hypertensive disease,
                    diabetes, cardiac or thyroid disease. Non-steroidal
                    anti-inflammatory agents (e.g. indomethacin) do
                    successfully suppress uterine contractions but there
                    is worry about premature closure of the ductus in
                    the infant and so they are not used routinely.
                    Dexamethasone is used to decrease the chance of
                    respiratory distress syndrome in the infant. Alcohol
                    has been used and is effective but has moderate
                    side effects. Pethidine is a sedative but will not stop
                    contractions.

3.29 A **False** Antepartum haemorrhage is defined as bleeding
      B **False** from the genital tract from 28 completed weeks of
      C **True**   pregnancy to the birth of the baby (therefore the
      D **True**   first and second stages of labour are included). It
      E **True**   occurs in approximately 3% of pregnancies. The
                    main causes are placenta praevia, placental
                    abruption, lesions of the cervix or vagina (including
                    carcinoma of the cervix), fetal and unexplained
                    causes. Fetal loss of blood, e.g. vasa praevia, is
                    uncommon and usually leads to significant fetal
                    distress for a small APH.

3.30 A **False** Placental abruption occurs after the 28th week and
      B **False** is called 'accidental' as opposed to the 'inevitable'
      C **True**   haemorrhage of placenta praevia. Postpartum
      D **False** haemorrhages are more common in women who
      E **True**   have had an antepartum haemorrhage. Beta-
                    adrenergics relax the uterus and make matters
                    worse by increasing the bleeding. The haemorrhage
                    may be revealed or totally concealed behind the
                    placenta.

3.31 A **True**   Severe abruption is dangerous to the mother. She
      B **True**   is frequently shocked and must be transfused,
      C **False** given analgesia and delivered rapidly. Caesarean
      D **True**   section is usually only indicated if the fetus is alive,
      E **True**   but may occasionally be performed to save the life
                    of the mother.

3.32 Complications of placental abruption include
A renal cortical necrosis
B eclampsia
C afibrinogenaemia
D disseminated intravascular coagulation
E intrauterine growth retardation

3.33 In placenta praevia
A all of the placenta is in the lower segment
B the fetal lie may be unstable
C life threatening haemorrhage may occur
D the fetus is often severely anaemic at birth
E bleeding rarely occurs before 36 weeks gestation

3.34 The following signs would support a diagnosis of placenta praevia
A a small uterus for the gestational age
B a transverse lie
C a tender uterus
D fetal heart rate decelerations
E uterine contractions

3.35 A woman with a known placenta praevia
A should be managed by examination under anaesthetic in theatre at 30 weeks gestation
B delivery should be by classical caesarean section if the placenta is anterior
C caesarean section should be performed by a consultant obstetrician
D at caesarean section postpartum haemorrhage is common
E is at a high risk of disseminated intravascular coagulation

(Answers overleaf)

3.32 A **True**   Severe abruption may lead to acute renal failure
    B **False**   and pituitary necrosis. Disseminated intravascular
    C **True**   coagulation occurs because of release of
    D **True**   thromboplastins from the uterus and this may
    E **True**   consume all of the circulating fibrinogen. Eclampsia
may cause these same complications, but is not
itself caused by an antepartum haemorrhage. In
less severe cases of abruption, when the pregnancy
continues, growth retardation may occur.

3.33 A **False**   For placenta praevia to be diagnosed, part of the
    B **True**   placenta must be in the lower segment of the
    C **True**   uterus. Because the lower pole of the uterus is
    D **False**   occupied the fetal lie is often unstable.
    E **False**   Haemorrhage from the placenta may be severe, and
this is why patients are kept in hospital. The blood
is maternal and not fetal. Patients frequently first
present between 30 and 34 weeks gestation.

3.34 A **False**   With a placenta praevia the bleeding is usually
    B **True**   painless, the abdomen is usually soft and
    C **False**   non-tender to palpation. Fetal parts are easily
    D **False**   palpable, the uterus is the right size for gestation
    E **False**   and there is not usually fetal distress unless the
mother becomes hypotensive.

3.35 A **False**   If a woman has a definite placenta praevia she
    B **False**   should be delivered by caesarean section. If there is
    C **True**   doubt about the diagnosis then some women are
    D **True**   managed by an examination in theatre at 38 weeks
    E **False**   gestation. It is a recommendation that caesarean
sections for placenta praevia should be carried out
by a consultant obstetrician, as the operation can
be quite hazardous. Most women who have an
anterior placenta praevia can still be delivered
safely by lower segment caesarean section but it is
occasionally an indication for a classical caesarean
section. Postpartum haemorrhage is common due
to the poor contractility of the lower segment. DIC
is associated with a placental abruption and not
placenta praevia.

3.36 A patient at 32 weeks gestation who has an antepartum haemorrhage

A requires admission to hospital
B requires placental localisation
C should be delivered forthwith
D should not be examined vaginally under any circumstances
E usually requires a blood transfusion

3.37 Intrauterine growth retardation may be suspected when

A polyhydramnios is present
B the uterus is small for dates
C fetal activity reduces at term
D maternal weight decreases
E serum oestriol levels fall

3.38 Symmetrical intrauterine growth retardation

A is usually caused by placental insufficiency
B is less worrying than asymmetrical intrauterine growth retardation
C is associated with oligohydramnios
D may be caused by excessive maternal alcohol ingestion
E may be caused by Potter's syndrome

3.39 The following methods of monitoring fetal well-being are of proven value

A kick charts
B biophysical profile
C Doppler study
D cardiotocography
E serum oestriol estimation

3.40 Fetal death in utero

A is more commonly associated with placenta praevia than abruption
B is a complication of diabetic pregnancy
C can be diagnosed on X-ray by the presence of Spalding's sign
D is sometimes associated with hypofibrinogenaemia
E is associated with polyhydramnios

(Answers overleaf)

3.36 A   **True**   The majority of haemorrhages at 32 weeks are
     B   **True**   fairly minor and do not warrant transfusion or
     C   **False**   delivery. They may be a sign of placenta praevia
     D   **False**   and ultrasound should be used to localise the
     E   **False**   placental site. Until this has been done, vaginal
                      examination should be avoided, unless the bleeding
                      is severe enough to call for immediate delivery in
                      which case examination in the operating theatre
                      can be performed.

3.37 A   **False**   Intrauterine growth retardation is associated with
     B   **True**   oligohydramnios, a small uterus and maternal
     C   **False**   weight loss and often with a fall in the values of
     D   **True**   placental function tests. Although it may be
     E   **True**   associated with diminished fetal movements, at
                      term virtually every fetus has reduced movements.

3.38 A   **False**   Intrauterine growth retardation may be symmetrical
     B   **False**   (decreased growth of the head circumference and
     C   **True**   abdominal circumference) or asymmetrical
     D   **True**   (decreased growth of the abdominal circumference
     E   **True**   with head circumference growth being spared).
                      Symmetrical intrauterine growth retardation has
                      many causes which include congenital
                      abnormalities, i.e. Potter's, congenital infections and
                      fetal alcohol syndrome. It is a worrying condition in
                      view of the common causes. Placental insufficiency
                      is usually associated with asymmetrical intrauterine
                      growth retardation, at least initially. Symmetrical or
                      asymmetrical intrauterine growth retardation is
                      associated with oligohydramnios.

3.39 A   **True**   Placental function tests can be clinical, biophysical
     B   **True**   or biochemical. Kick charts, biophysical profile,
     C   **True**   doppler studies, cardiotocography and ultrasound
     D   **True**   estimation of growth are of proven value.
     E   **False**   Biochemical tests such as serum oestriol estimation
                      are of no proven value.

3.40 A   **False**   Abruption leads to separation of the placenta from
     B   **True**   the uterus and frequently causes fetal death.
     C   **True**   Sudden fetal death in late pregnancy occurs in
     D   **True**   diabetic pregnancies. Spalding's sign is overlapping
     E   **False**   of the fetal skull bones and appears a few days
                      after death. Fetal death leads to oligohydramnios
                      and if the products are not removed may lead to
                      hypofibrinogenaemia.

3.41 Disseminated intravascular coagulation (DIC) is associated with
- A   pre-eclamptic toxaemia
- B   placental abruption
- C   amniotic fluid embolism
- D   hydatidiform mole
- E   intrauterine fetal death

3.42 Rhesus disease in the fetus
- A   is due to maternal anti-D
- B   can be prevented by anti-D
- C   occurs commonly in the firstborn of Rhesus negative women
- D   occurs in Rhesus negative offspring of Rhesus positive mothers
- E   can be treated by intrauterine transfusion

3.43 The grand multiparous patient is more at risk of
- A   varicose veins of the legs
- B   iron deficiency anaemia
- C   operative delivery
- D   face presentation
- E   cord prolapse

3.44 A high head at term could be due to
- A   fundal fibroid
- B   wrong dates
- C   placental abruption
- D   cephalopelvic disproportion
- E   occipitoposterior position

3.45 Postmaturity
- A   is defined as a pregnancy which has extended beyond 41 completed weeks of pregnancy
- B   is an indication for induction of labour
- C   is associated with a higher incidence of meconium in labour
- D   is associated with bigger babies than babies born at 40 weeks
- E   at 42 weeks is associated with a higher perinatal mortality rate than a baby born at 40 weeks gestation

(Answers overleaf)

3.41 A **True**   Pre-eclamptic toxaemia, placental abruption,
      B **True**   amniotic fluid embolism, hydatidiform mole and
      C **True**   IUFD are all associated with disseminated
      D **True**   intravascular coagulation. In all of these conditions
      E **True**   a clotting screen should be a routine investigation.
                    Treatment involves close liaison with and advice
                    from the doctors in the haematology department.

3.42 A **True**   Rhesus disease occurs when a Rhesus negative
      B **True**   woman is immunised against Rhesus positive red
      C **False** blood cells (usually in a previous pregnancy), forms
      D **False** anti-D which crosses into the Rhesus positive fetus
      E **True**   and causes anaemia. Injection of the mother with
                    anti-D after pregnancy will destroy fetal red cells
                    and prevent immunisation. Once a fetus is affected
                    treatment is by intrauterine transfusion and early
                    delivery.

3.43 A **True**   A grand multipara is in her sixth or subsequent
      B **True**   pregnancy. Iron deficiency anaemia is common and
      C **True**   varicose veins of the legs tend to worsen with each
      D **True**   pregnancy. The lower ratio of uterine muscle to
      E **True**   fibrous tissue makes unstable lie, malpresentation,
                    malposition, cord prolapse, uterine rupture and
                    operative delivery more likely.

3.44 A **False** In a primigravid patient the fetal head engages
      B **True**   from 36 weeks gestation. In multiparous patients
      C **False** the head may not engage until labour is
      D **True**   commenced. A high head at term may be found
      E **True**   because of wrong dates or for fetal or maternal
                    reasons. The fetus may be too big (hydrocephaly or
                    cephalopelvic disproportion) or present with a
                    larger diameter (occipitoposterior position). There
                    may be something else in the pelvis (the placenta,
                    fibroids in the lower part of the uterus, ovarian
                    masses, full bladder and full rectum).

3.45 A **False** Term is defined as a gestation of 37 to 42 weeks
      B **False** and postmaturity is after 42 completed weeks of
      C **True**   pregnancy. At 42 weeks gestation the perinatal
      D **True**   mortality rate is no higher than at 40 weeks
      E **False** gestation and provided that there are no other
                    indications for delivery, induction of labour for this
                    reason alone is not necessary. There is, however, a
                    higher incidence of meconium in labour, less
                    moulding of the fetal skull and a higher average
                    birthweight than babies born at 40 weeks.

3.46 The management of a woman with pregnancy-induced hypertension at 36 weeks gestation includes
- A   admission to hospital
- B   ultrasound scan
- C   a serum urate estimation
- D   treatment with oral anti-hypertensive medication
- E   administration of aspirin

3.47 In pregnancy-induced hypertension
- A   the patient is normotensive before 28 weeks gestation
- B   the patient has significant proteinuria, a loss of 300 mg per 24 hours or more in the urine
- C   the patient is usually primigravid
- D   the end point for the diastolic pressure should be taken as Korotkoff IV
- E   the patient more commonly is a smoker than a non-smoker

3.48 Symptoms and signs of pre-eclampsia include
- A   epigastric pain
- B   vomiting
- C   fits
- D   hypo-reflexia
- E   oliguria

3.49 Severe pre-eclampsia may be complicated by
- A   rupture of the liver
- B   intrauterine growth retardation
- C   temporary loss of sight
- D   cardiovascular accidents
- E   intrauterine fetal death

3.50 Pre-eclampsia is accompanied by
- A   disseminated intravascular coagulation
- B   reduced blood flow to the placental bed
- C   swelling of glomeruli
- D   a fall in plasma urate concentration
- E   thrombocytopenia

(Answers overleaf)

3.46 A **False** Most women with pregnancy-induced hypertension
     B **True**   can be managed as an out-patient either with
     C **True**   monitoring by the district midwife or on a
     D **False** pregnancy assessment unit. Pregnancy-induced
     E **False** hypertension can be associated with intrauterine
                  growth retardation and so an ultrasound scan
                  should be performed. A serum urate estimation can
                  be an indicator of the onset of pre-eclamptic
                  toxaemia. At 36 weeks there is no advantage to
                  treatment with anti-hypertensives or aspirin.

3.47 A **False** Pregnancy-induced hypertension is defined as
     B **False** hypertension occurring in women who have been
     C **True**   normotensive before 20 weeks gestation. It is
     D **True**   predominantly a disease of primigravida. Smokers
     E **False** have approximately half the risk of non-smokers of
                  developing the disease. In pregnancy, when taking
                  the blood pressure, muffled sounds may be heard
                  all the way down to 0 mmHg, so Korotkoff IV is
                  taken as the end point.

3.48 A **True**   In severe pre-eclampsia oedema and haemorrhages
     B **True**   under the capsule of the liver cause epigastric pain.
     C **False** Vomiting may occur. Renal function deteriorates
     D **False** and the intravascular volume falls leading to
     E **True**   oliguria. Hyper-reflexia occurs, when fits have
                  begun the patient has eclampsia.

3.49 A **True**   Severe pre-eclampsia can be complicated by
     B **True**   disseminated intravascular coagulation and
     C **True**   haemorrhage in maternal organs. Periportal and
     D **True**   subcapsular haemorrhages in the liver may lead to
     E **True**   liver rupture. In the brain there may be cerebro-
                  vascular haemorrhages. In the eye there may be
                  retinal detachment, oedema and thrombosis
                  leading to blindness in up to 2% of cases (usually
                  temporary). Placental function decreases and
                  growth retardation or fetal death can occur.

3.50 A **True**   Pre-eclampsia is a multi-system disease that is
     B **True**   characterised by disseminated intravascular
     C **True**   coagulation (usually mild) and thrombocytopenia,
     D **False** failure of the second wave of trophoblast invasion
     E **True**   with consequent retention of spiral artery muscle
                  and reduced blood flow in the uterus. In the kidney
                  there is thickening of the epithelium and the
                  endothelial cells swell. Plasma uric acid
                  concentration increases.

3.51 Amniotic fluid embolism

A   is a complication of the puerperium
B   is complicated by disseminated intravascular coagulation
C   causes cyanosis
D   causes bronchospasm
E   leads to maternal death in 30% of cases

3.52 Gross obesity in a pregnant patient causes an increase in the incidence of

A   leg oedema
B   malpresentation
C   hypertension
D   cephalopelvic disproportion
E   multiple pregnancy

3.53 Concerning HIV infection and pregnancy

A   termination of pregnancy should be offered
B   breast feeding is absolutely contraindicated
C   babies should be delivered by caesarean section
D   HIV antibody testing of the newborn child accurately determines the chance of it being affected
E   the infant will be affected in 50% of cases

3.54 The risks of premature rupture of the membranes include

A   development of premature labour
B   cord prolapse
C   fetal pneumonia
D   placental abruption
E   maternal septicaemia

(Answers overleaf)

3.51 A   **False**   Amniotic fluid embolism is a major obstetric
      B   **True**   emergency which is estimated to lead to maternal
      C   **True**   death in up to 95% of cases, although it is difficult
      D   **False**   to confirm the diagnosis if the patient survives. It
      E   **False**   occurs during labour or occasionally at caesarean
                        section when amniotic fluid enters the maternal
                        circulation, causing platelet and fibrin thrombi to
                        lodge in the lungs leading to respiratory distress
                        and cyanosis. DIC and hypofibrinogenaemia occur.
                        Bronchospasm is a complication of aspiration.

3.52 A   **True**   The obese pregnant patient has an increased risk of
      B   **False**   developing hypertensive disorders. She frequently
      C   **True**   has leg oedema. As the fetus is often large,
      D   **True**   cephalopelvic disproportion and shoulder dystocia
      E   **False**   are more common. Malpresentations and multiple
                        pregnancy are no more common, but are more
                        difficult to detect.

3.53 A   **True**   Perinatal transmission of HIV infection occurs in
      B   **False**   5–30% of pregnancies. The infection is usually
      C   **False**   passed to the fetus transplacentally but can also be
      D   **False**   transmitted in breast milk. It is generally thought
      E   **False**   that if the fetus is to be affected it is more likely to
                        be affected transplacentally than via breast milk.
                        There is, however, a high risk of passing the virus
                        to a fetus during breast feeding if the mother
                        becomes HIV positive in the puerperium. Direct
                        spread from the genital tract has also been
                        implicated as a possible source of viral infection for
                        the fetus. This, however, still does not mean that
                        the baby should be born by caesarean section as
                        this in itself may carry potential hazards. The time
                        required for elimination of passively transmitted
                        IgG from the mother will affect the significance of
                        HIV antibody testing in the newborn. Comparison of
                        maternal and fetal antibody and sequential
                        antibody tests are necessary to reach a more
                        accurate diagnosis.

3.54 A   **True**   The risks are of premature labour, malpresentation
      B   **True**   and cord prolapse and ascending infection affecting
      C   **True**   the mother and fetus. Management is a balance
      D   **False**   between prematurity and infection.
      E   **True**

3.55 **Maternal smoking in pregnancy is associated with**
 A   low birthweight infants
 B   spontaneous abortion
 C   an increased perinatal mortality
 D   sudden infant death syndrome in early childhood
 E   placental abruption

3.56 **Assessment of fetal maturity can be performed by**
 A   ultrasound scan at 16 weeks
 B   X-ray of the fetal knee at 30 weeks
 C   bimanual examination at 10 weeks
 D   examination of fetal cells in amniotic fluid at term
 E   measurement of human placental lactogen at 32 weeks

3.57 **An unstable lie is associated with**
 A   prematurity
 B   placenta praevia
 C   uterus didelphys
 D   a fundal fibroid
 E   grand multiparity

3.58 **Breech presentation is associated with**
 A   prematurity
 B   polyhydramnios
 C   oligohydramnios
 D   hydrocephaly
 E   anencephaly

3.59 **A frank or extended breech is**
 A   easily turned by external cephalic version
 B   the commonest type of breech presentation in
     primigravidae
 C   less likely than a flexed breech to be complicated by a
     cord prolapse
 D   the presentation in approximately 2% of women near term
 E   sometimes known as a footling

3.60 **External cephalic version is contraindicated in patients with**
 A   an antepartum haemorrhage
 B   placenta praevia
 C   multiple pregnancy
 D   hypertension
 E   a scarred uterus

(Answers overleaf)

3.55 A **True** There is an increase in spontaneous abortion, low
 B **True** birthweight babies, placental abruption and
 C **True** perinatal mortality rate in women who smoke.
 D **True** Sudden infant death syndrome has a peak
 E **True** incidence at about 2–4 months and is about 1.5
 times more likely in a child whose mother has
 smoked during her pregnancy.

3.56 A **True** Gestation can be determined by ultrasound
 B **False** measurement of biparietal diameter before 30
 C **True** weeks, clinical assessment of uterine size early in
 D **True** pregnancy or X-ray demonstration of the epiphyses
 E **False** at the lower femur at 36 weeks and the upper tibia
 at 38–40 weeks. At term 50% of the cells should
 stain orange with nile blue sulphate. HPL values
 vary so much that a single measurement is of no
 value.

3.57 A **True** When the fetus is premature the ratio of the liquor
 B **True** to fetus is greater and fetal mobility is greater. A
 C **False** uterus with poor tone (multiparity) or with a mass
 D **False** in the pelvis (placenta praevia) will also cause
 E **True** instability. Cervical, but not fundal fibroids cause
 instability. A double uterus will function normally,
 possibly with a greater incidence of persistent
 breech presentations because of the lack of room
 for the fetus to turn round.

3.58 A **True** 25% of fetuses present by the breech at 30 weeks,
 B **True** but only 3% at term. Fetal abnormalities such as
 C **True** hydrocephaly and anencephaly often present by the
 D **True** breech because of the better fit in the pelvis.
 E **True** Polyhydramnios and oligohydramnios are
 associated with fetal abnormality, but also make the
 fetus too mobile and immobile respectively,
 increasing the incidence of breech presentation.

3.59 A **False** An extended breech has its legs splinting its body,
 B **True** with flexed hips and extended knees. It is very
 C **True** difficult to turn because of this splinting effect. It is
 D **True** the commonest breech presentation. A footling has
 E **False** one leg extended and one leg flexed, presenting
 with a single foot first.

3.60 A **True** Leaving aside the advisability of performing an ECV
 B **True** at all, in these cases there is either a risk to the
 C **True** mother, of placental separation or uterine rupture,
 D **True** or it is pointless because caesarean section would
 E **True** be undertaken anyway.

MEDICAL DISORDERS IN PREGNANCY

3.61 Patients with rheumatic heart disease who become pregnant
  A   should always be given iron and folate supplements
  B   commonly develop atrial fibrillation
  C   frequently develop pre-eclampsia
  D   should have operative procedures covered by prophylactic antibiotics
  E   usually remain asymptomatic

3.62 The following maternal conditions significantly increase fetal loss
  A   Fallot's tetralogy
  B   mitral stenosis
  C   uncorrected coarctation of the aorta
  D   pulmonary hypertension
  E   heart block

3.63 Essential hypertension in pregnancy is
  A   usually diagnosed in the third trimester
  B   commonly associated with a strong family history of cardiovascular problems
  C   usually associated with marked proteinuria
  D   usually asymptomatic
  E   more common in women over the age of 35

3.64 Patients with uncomplicated essential hypertension in pregnancy
  A   will develop pre-eclampsia more commonly than normotensive women
  B   have a very high risk of developing antepartum haemorrhage
  C   have a normal serum uric acid concentration
  D   should be offered therapeutic abortion
  E   frequently become normotensive in the second trimester

3.65 The following drugs are of use in treating essential hypertension in pregnancy
  A   frusemide
  B   methyldopa
  C   labetalol
  D   atenolol
  E   angiotensin-converting-enzyme inhibitors

(Answers overleaf)

MEDICAL DISORDERS IN PREGNANCY

3.61 A   **True**   The haemodynamic changes of pregnancy increase
     B   **False**   the strain on the heart. Anaemia will exacerbate
     C   **False**   this. Atrial fibrillation is present in less than 3% of
     D   **True**   cases. These patients frequently manage well and
     E   **True**   remain asymptomatic, they are not at any extra risk
                     of hypertensive disorders. Operative procedures
                     should be covered by antibiotics to prevent
                     development of bacterial endocarditis.

3.62 A   **True**   Patients with rheumatic heart disease such as mitral
     B   **False**   stenosis generally do well in pregnancy. Pulmonary
     C   **True**   hypertension and cyanotic heart disease, as is seen
     D   **True**   in Fallot's tetralogy, lead to increased maternal and
     E   **False**   fetal loss. Coarctation of the aorta leads to poor
                     placental perfusion and increased fetal death rates.
                     Heart block in the mother does not seem to affect
                     the fetus.

3.63 A   **False**   Hypertension appearing in the third trimester is
     B   **True**   usually assumed to be pregnancy-induced rather
     C   **False**   than essential. Essential hypertension is associated
     D   **True**   with a positive family history, increases with age
     E   **True**   and is usually asymptomatic. Proteinuria usually
                     denotes pre-eclampsia or renal disease.

3.64 A   **True**   Patients who are hypertensive in the first trimester
     B   **False**   of pregnancy frequently have lower blood pressure
     C   **True**   in the second trimester. They develop pre-
     D   **False**   eclampsia more frequently, but are not particularly
     E   **True**   at risk of antepartum haemorrhage unless the
                     hypertension is very severe. Pre-eclamptics
                     frequently have raised uric acid levels, essential
                     hypertensives do not. It is not an indication for
                     abortion.

3.65 A   **False**   Diuretics should be avoided because of their effects
     B   **True**   when pre-eclampsia is superadded. Methyldopa
     C   **True**   and labetalol have both been extensively used and
     D   **False**   are safe and effective. Atenolol is associated with
     E   **False**   intrauterine growth retardation and angiotensin-
                     converting-enzyme inhibitors have been implicated
                     in intrauterine fetal deaths in sheep, so have not
                     been used in pregnancy in humans.

3.66 In labour, a patient with essential hypertension

A   should not be given epidural anaesthesia
B   can safely be given intravenous Syntocinon
C   should not be given Syntometrine as a routine in the third stage of labour
D   needs sedation with diazepam
E   should be treated with hydralazine

3.67 Pregnant patients with a past history of deep venous thrombosis should be

A   anticoagulated with heparin throughout pregnancy and the puerperium
B   treated with warfarin in the second and third trimesters
C   warfarinised in the puerperium
D   only anticoagulated if the previous deep venous thrombosis occurred in a pregnancy
E   delivered by elective caesarean section

3.68 Venous thrombosis associated with pregnancy

A   is an uncommon diagnosis in the antenatal period
B   is more dangerous antenatally than in the puerperium
C   requires treatment with warfarin in labour
D   is frequently asymptomatic
E   should not be treated until after the patient has been delivered

3.69 Autoimmune idiopathic thrombocytopenic purpura in pregnancy

A   gets better
B   may cause fetal thrombocytopenia
C   should be treated by splenectomy
D   is treated with steroids
E   is treated with intravenous IgG

3.70 The risk of thromboembolism in pregnancy and the puerperium is increased

A   by increasing maternal age
B   in primigravidae
C   by the presence of lupus anticoagulant
D   by excess of circulating antithrombin III
E   after caesarean section

(Answers overleaf)

3.66 A **False** There is no contraindication to intravenous
 B **True** Syntocinon or epidural anaesthesia in these
 C **True** patients. Diazepam will not make the patient
 D **False** normotensive and will depress the neonate.
 E **False** Syntometrine or ergometrine may precipitate heart
 failure or increase blood pressure and should be
 avoided, Syntocinon being preferred. Hydralazine is
 used for the control of severe hypertension, usually
 in pre-eclamptics.

3.67 A **False** A past history of DVT is a significant risk factor for
 B **False** developing thromboembolism in a pregnancy.
 C **True** There is no difference between those who have had
 D **False** a DVT in a previous pregnancy, taking a combined
 E **False** oral contraceptive preparation or coincidentally. The
 risk of anticoagulation, fetal effects with warfarin
 and maternal osteoporosis with long term heparin,
 are such that prophylaxis should be avoided in
 pregnancy except in special circumstances
 (recurrent DVTs, antithrombin III deficiency). It is
 best to warfarinise the patient in the puerperium
 when she is at most risk. Caesarean section adds to
 the risks and is only performed for obstetric
 reasons.

3.68 A **True** Venous thrombosis usually follows delivery. In the
 B **True** antenatal period it is uncommon, frequently
 C **False** asymptomatic, often missed and therefore very
 D **True** dangerous. It must always be treated immediately
 E **False** with heparin. Warfarin crosses the placenta and
 anticoagulates the fetus and may cause bleeding at
 delivery. Also, warfarin cannot easily or rapidly be
 reversed (unlike heparin) and a warfarinised woman
 is at significant risk of haemorrhage in labour.

3.69 A **False** ITP gets worse in pregnancy. The circulating IgG
 B **True** crosses to the fetus and may lead to destruction of
 C **False** fetal platelets. This can be avoided by treating the
 D **True** patient with intravenous IgG which reduces platelet
 E **True** destruction. Treatment with steroids is also
 successful, but splenectomy is to be avoided
 because of an associated increase in maternal
 mortality.

3.70 A **True** Increasing age and parity are risk factors for
 B **False** thromboembolism, as are the presence of lupus
 C **True** anticoagulant and antithrombin III deficiency. One
 D **False** of the major factors in promoting
 E **True** thromboembolism in the puerperium, when the
 patient is at most risk, is caesarean section.

3.71 In severe disseminated intravascular coagulation
  A   fibrin degradation product levels are raised
  B   the uterus is often relaxed
  C   treatment is initiated with heparin
  D   hypofibrinogenaemia occurs
  E   thrombocytopenia occurs

3.72 Disseminated intravascular coagulation in pregnancy is a complication of
  A   placental abruption
  B   essential hypertension
  C   eclampsia
  D   epilepsy
  E   aseptic abortion

3.73 Patients with sickle-cell disease
  A   should have their pregnancies terminated
  B   are at greater risk of spontaneous abortion
  C   commonly go into premature labour
  D   should have blood transfusions at six-weekly intervals in pregnancy
  E   are of greatest risk of sickling in labour

3.74 Beta-thalassaemia
  A   is only seen in patients of Mediterranean origin
  B   is inherited as an autosomal recessive
  C   in pregnancy is treated with parenteral iron
  D   minor does not lead to complications in pregnancy
  E   major is compatible with pregnancy

3.75 Pregnant patients taking anticonvulsant therapy
  A   have an increased risk of congenital abnormalities
  B   have an increased risk of premature delivery
  C   should not be given folate supplements
  D   deliver neonates that may have bleeding disorders
  E   have a high incidence of megaloblastic anaemia

(Answers overleaf)

3.71 A **True**   In severe DIC much of the circulating fibrinogen,
      B **True**   clotting factors and platelets are consumed.
      C **False**   Fibrinolysis also occurs and FDP levels are raised
      D **True**   which in turn inhibit myometrial contraction, often
      E **True**   causing uterine haemorrhage. Heparinisation is not
                     appropriate, treatment involves replacing clotting
                     factors (using fresh frozen plasma) and platelets
                     and removing the initiating problem.

3.72 A **True**   DIC is secondary to a variety of pathological events
      B **False**   in pregnancy, including pre-eclampsia, eclampsia,
      C **True**   abruption, amniotic fluid embolism, septic abortion
      D **False**   and severe haemorrhage. Unless proteinuric
      E **True**   pregnancy-induced hypertension complicates
                     essential hypertension, DIC will not occur. It is the
                     eclamptic process, not the fits themselves that
                     cause DIC and epileptic fits are not associated with
                     the condition.

3.73 A **False**   With modern management maternal and perinatal
      B **True**   morbidity and mortality have been considerably
      C **True**   reduced. These patients are at risk of spontaneous
      D **True**   abortion, premature labour and intrauterine growth
      E **True**   retardation and particularly a sickling crisis when
                     oxygenation and hydration are compromised such
                     as in labour. Regular transfusions reduce the
                     concentration of HbS present and reduce the risks
                     of pregnancy to mother and fetus.

3.74 A **False**   Beta-thalassaemia is found in Mediterranean people
      B **True**   and Asians. It is inherited as an autosomal
      C **False**   recessive, homozygotes having thalassaemia major
      D **False**   and heterozygotes thalassaemia minor. Patients
      E **False**   with thalassaemia minor develop anaemia in
                     pregnancy. They require oral iron and folate but
                     should not be given parenteral iron as the major
                     danger in thalassaemia is iron overload leading to
                     multiple organ damage. Successful pregnancy is
                     uncommon in thalassaemia major but is described.
                     With more modern treatment it is likely to become
                     more common in affected populations.

3.75 A **True**   Anticonvulsant drugs cause folate deficiency which
      B **True**   is exacerbated in pregnancy and may lead to
      C **False**   megaloblastic anaemia and bleeding diatheses in
      D **True**   the neonate. The risks of premature labour, low
      E **True**   birth weight and congenital abnormality are
                     increased. Folate supplements are not
                     contraindicated.

3.76 In pregnancy

    A   serum folate levels fall

    B   folic acid deficiency leads to microcytic anaemia

    C   macrocytic anaemia is usually due to vitamin B_{12} deficiency

    D   fetal malformations are less common if serum folic acid levels are high

    E   folic acid supplements should always be given to women carrying twins

3.77 In the management of iron deficiency anaemia in pregnancy

    A   oral iron therapy usually leads to diarrhoea

    B   the treated patient's haemoglobin concentration will increase by 2 g/dl per week

    C   the haematological response to intramuscular iron therapy is faster than that following oral therapy

    D   200 mg of iron taken orally each day is adequate

    E   total dose infusion of iron is contraindicated

3.78 The asthmatic pregnant patient's

    A   fetus will usually be growth retarded

    B   respiratory problems will worsen during her pregnancy

    C   treatment can safely include corticosteroids

    D   treatment can safely include salbutamol

    E   labour can be induced using PGE_2 or PGF2α

3.79 The following drugs can be used safely to treat the pregnant woman with tuberculosis

    A   rifampicin

    B   isoniazid

    C   ethambutol

    D   streptomycin

    E   ethionamide

3.80 Concerning thyrotoxicosis in pregnancy

    A   most cases are newly diagnosed in pregnancy

    B   most cases are due to Graves' disease

    C   there is frequently a family history of thyroid disease

    D   the disease is made worse by pregnancy

    E   fetal thyrotoxicosis may occur

(Answers overleaf)

3.76 A **True**   In pregnancy renal clearance of folate is doubled
      B **False** and there may be decreased absorption from the
      C **False** gut. In addition, the fetus requires folate. Untreated,
      D **True**   maternal serum folate concentration will fall.
      E **True**   Deficiency will eventually lead to megaloblastic
               anaemia, B_{12} deficiency is uncommon in this age
               group. Folate supplements given to women before
               pregnancy and during the first trimester decrease
               the congenital fetal abnormality rate, particularly in
               respect of CNS abnormalities. In multiple
               pregnancy folate deficiency is exacerbated.

3.77 A **False** Oral iron therapy usually leads to constipation. The
      B **False** speed of the haematological response is the same
      C **False** regardless of the route of administration, being
      D **True**   approximately 1 g/dl per week. Although
      E **False** anaphylatic reactions to total dose infusion may
               occur, as long as a small test dose is given the
               procedure is safe.

3.78 A **False** Asthma is a very common condition in women of
      B **False** reproductive age. Pregnancy has no consistent
      C **True**   effect upon the disease, and, except in a few cases
      D **True**   of severe disease, the fetus is not affected.
      E **False** Salbutamol and corticosteroids have been used
               extensively in pregnancy without ill effects.
               Prostaglandins, particularly $PGF2\alpha$, are broncho-
               constrictor and should be avoided.

3.79 A **False** Pulmonary tuberculosis has been an uncommon
      B **True**   condition in the general population for some years,
      C **True**   but is now once again on the increase and may be
      D **False** found in pregnant women. Ethionamide is
      E **False** teratogenic and rifampicin causes variable severe
               fetal abnormalities. Streptomycin causes fetal
               eighth nerve damage. Ethambutol is safe in
               pregnancy. Isoniazid may cause CNS abnormalities,
               but this risk is lessened by the patient taking
               pyridoxine concurrently.

3.80 A **False** Most cases of thyroid disease in pregnancy are due
      B **True**   to Graves' disease and have been diagnosed before
      C **True**   the pregnancy began. In approximately 50% of
      D **False** cases there is a relevant family history. The disease
      E **True**   is generally not affected by pregnancy, but
               untreated it will increase the rate of abortion and
               premature labour. In some cases antibodies enter
               the fetus and stimulate the fetal thyroid.

3.81 In pregnancy, appropriate treatments for thyrotoxicosis include
- A   termination of pregnancy
- B   carbimazole
- C   partial thyroidectomy
- D   propranolol
- E   radioactive iodine

3.82 Hashimoto's disease in pregnancy
- A   increases the spontaneous abortion rate
- B   increases the stillbirth rate
- C   responds to thyroxine
- D   causes deafness
- E   may lead to transient hypothyroidism in the neonate

3.83 In pregnancy, pituitary prolactinomas
- A   cause galactorrhoea
- B   shrink
- C   are associated with diabetes insipidus
- D   may cause bitemporal hemianopia
- E   are an indication to perform elective caesarean section

3.84 Diabetes insipidus
- A   does not affect fertility
- B   is an indication for termination of pregnancy
- C   is made worse by pregnancy
- D   causes postmaturity
- E   does not affect lactation

3.85 Addison's disease
- A   is made worse by pregnancy
- B   is an indication for termination of pregnancy
- C   is an indication for elective caesarean section
- D   has no effect upon the fetus
- E   now carries a good prognosis in pregnancy

(Answers overleaf)

3.81　A　**False**　Thyrotoxicosis can be adequately controlled in
　　　B　**True**　pregnancy and it is not an indication for
　　　C　**True**　termination of pregnancy. Carbimazole is safe,
　　　D　**True**　although the lowest possible dose should be used
　　　E　**False**　to minimise effects upon the fetus. Propranolol is
effective, the risk of intrauterine growth retardation
being more theoretical than real (atenolol does
cause IUGR). Radioactive iodine will destroy the
fetal thyroid and must not be given. If medical
treatment fails or the goitre is large enough to
cause obstructive symptoms then partial
thyroidectomy is indicated, best performed in the
second trimester.

3.82　A　**True**　In hypothyroidism due to Hashimoto's disease the
　　　B　**True**　abortion and stillbirth rates are doubled. Antibodies
　　　C　**True**　enter the fetus and may cause transient neonatal
　　　D　**False**　problems. Deafness and mental retardation are
　　　E　**True**　features of iodine deficiency in the first trimester.

3.83　A　**False**　Prolactinomas enlarge in pregnancy and may press
　　　B　**False**　on the optic chiasma causing bitemporal
　　　C　**True**　hemianopia. Pressure on the posterior pituitary may
　　　D　**True**　occasionally cause diabetes insipidus. Despite the
　　　E　**False**　high prolactin concentration, the high oestrogen
concentration of pregnancy prevents galactorrhoea.
Labour progresses normally.

3.84　A　**True**　Fertility, pregnancy, delivery and lactation are
　　　B　**False**　unaffected by diabetes insipidus. The condition is
　　　C　**True**　made worse by pregnancy and fetal pituitary ADH
　　　D　**False**　does not help.
　　　E　**True**

3.85　A　**True**　Addison's disease used to cause significant
　　　B　**False**　maternal mortality, but the prognosis is now much
　　　C　**False**　better. Vomiting and electrolyte loss, the stress of
　　　D　**True**　labour and diuresis in the puerperium combined to
　　　E　**True**　aggravate the condition. The fetus is unaffected.
Caesarean section is performed for obstetric
indications.

3.86 Serum fructosamine concentration
- A   is dependent upon haemoglobin concentration
- B   is dependent upon plasma protein concentration
- C   falls in pregnancy
- D   is a useful guide to current blood glucose concentration
- E   is a useful guide to blood glucose concentrations in the recent past

3.87 In diabetic pregnancies
- A   congenital abnormalities are commoner
- B   insulin requirements increase
- C   intrauterine growth retardation is common
- D   oligohydramnios occurs
- E   monilial vaginitis is common

3.88 In a pregnant, insulin-requiring diabetic the following changes are irreversible
- A   worsening of retinopathy
- B   hypertension
- C   worsening of renal disease
- D   increase in insulin requirements
- E   atherosclerosis in uterine spiral arteries

3.89 In a pregnant patient with diabetes mellitus
- A   glycosuria is a reliable sign of poor control
- B   the blood glucose should be maintained at approximately 9 mmol/l
- C   persistent hyperglycaemia is worse than occasional hypoglycaemia
- D   all patients should be admitted to hospital to establish tight control of the blood sugar concentration
- E   patients must be delivered by 38 weeks gestation

3.90 In the neonatal period the child of a diabetic is more prone to develop
- A   hyperglycaemia
- B   respiratory distress syndrome
- C   anaemia
- D   hypocalcaemia
- E   jaundice

(Answers overleaf)

3.86 A **False**   Serum fructosamine is not dependent on
      B **True**   haemoglobin concentration and consequently is a
      C **True**   more stable and useful substance to measure in
      D **False**   diabetic pregnancies than glycosylated
      E **True**   haemoglobin. It is dependent upon plasma protein
                     concentration, and it falls in pregnancy, but this is a
                     reasonably stable event for a given pregnancy. As
                     with glycosylated haemoglobin it reflects long term
                     rather than current blood glucose concentration.

3.87 A **True**   Pregnancy is diabetogenic and insulin requirements
      B **True**   invariably increase. Unless the patient is
      C **False**   exceptionally well-controlled before the pregnancy
      D **False**   the congenital abnormality rate is increased,
      E **True**   particularly cardiac and CNS abnormalities.
                     Although IUGR can occur, particularly if the
                     pregnancy is complicated by pregnancy induced
                     hypertension, macrosomia is commoner.
                     Polyhydramnios occurs in some cases. Infection
                     with *Candida albicans* is common.

3.88 A **True**   Although all of these changes take place to a
      B **False**   greater or lesser extent in pregnancy, they are all
      C **False**   reversible with the exception of diabetic
      D **False**   proliferative retinopathy. It is for this reason that
      E **False**   known diabetics must be investigated for
                     retinopathy and treated if it is found early in the
                     pregnancy.

3.89 A **False**   Because of the increased glomerular filtration rate,
      B **False**   glycosuria is common in pregnancy and is an
      C **True**   unreliable measure of blood glucose concentration.
      D **False**   Blood sugar should ideally be kept below 7 mmol/l.
      E **False**   Transient hypoglycaemia has little effect on
                     pregnancy. Management is at home; when patients
                     are admitted they become more difficult to control
                     because of the alteration in their activity levels. The
                     object is to avoid iatrogenic prematurity and with
                     good control delivery should be after 38 weeks.

3.90 A **False**   Hyperinsulinaemia and profound hypoglycaemia
      B **True**   may occur. Respiratory distress syndrome occurs
      C **False**   more frequently, even in babies delivered near
      D **True**   term. Insulin increases the release of erythropoietin
      E **True**   and polycythaemia may occur. Hypocalcaemia is
                     common. Jaundice is more common because of
                     prematurity, polycythaemia and bruising if a
                     macrosomic infant is delivered vaginally.

3.91 **The following organisms, when acquired at birth, cause conjunctivitis in the neonate**
    A human wart (papilloma) virus
    B *Neisseria gonorrhoeae*
    C *Herpes simplex type II*
    D *Chlamydia trachomatis*
    E *Trichomonas vaginalis*

3.92 **In rubella infection in pregnancy**
    A the incubation period is 7–10 days
    B in the first 10 weeks of pregnancy the risk of congenital abnormality is 90%
    C after 16 weeks the risk of congenital anomaly is 50%
    D fetal pulmonary artery hypoplasia is common
    E intrauterine growth retardation is a common complication

3.93 **The following vaccines should not be used in pregnancy**
    A measles
    B influenza
    C mumps
    D hepatitis B
    E poliomyelitis

3.94 **Listeria monocytogenes infection in pregnancy**
    A is frequently centred on the urinary tract
    B is teratogenic
    C is transmitted to the fetus
    D increases the abortion and premature delivery rates
    E causes meningo-encephalitis in the neonate

3.95 **Viral hepatitis A in pregnancy**
    A occurs in the same frequency as in non-pregnant patients
    B frequently causes spontaneous abortion
    C is not an indication for termination of pregnancy
    D may cause acute hepatic necrosis
    E may produce a viraemia in the fetus

3.96 **Causes of generalised pruritus in pregnancy include**
    A trichomoniasis
    B herpes gestationis
    C scabies infestation
    D diabetes mellitus
    E syphilis

(Answers overleaf)

3.91 A **False** *Trichomonas vaginalis* does not affect the fetus.
      B **True**   The neonate may be infected with the wart virus
      C **True**   and may develop laryngeal or tracheal polyps, but
      D **True**   not conjunctivitis. The other agents can all be
      E **False** acquired during passage through the birth canal
                    and cause conjunctivitis.

3.92 A **False** The incubation period for rubella is 14–21 days. The
      B **True**   risk of infection causing a congenital anomaly falls
      C **False** from 90% in the first 10 weeks to less than 10%
      D **True**   after 16 weeks. Very common sequelae are
      E **True**   pulmonary artery hypoplasia, intrauterine growth
                    retardation and hepatosplenomegaly.

3.93 A **True**   Live vaccines are contraindicated in pregnancy and
      B **False** examples include measles, mumps, poliomyelitis
      C **True**   and rubella. Inactivated vaccines such as influenza
      D **False** and hepatitis B are safe to use if there is a
      E **True**   significant risk of infection or it would be
                    particularly dangerous for the woman to become
                    infected.

3.94 A **True**   Listeria infection in pregnancy is usually urinary. If
      B **False** the infection is transmitted to the fetus it leads to
      C **True**   intrauterine death, abortion or premature labour. If
      D **True**   the baby is alive at birth it usually has meningo-
      E **True**   encephalitis and will die shortly afterwards.
                    Transmission of infection may occur in labour from
                    the vagina, again leading to encephalitis.

3.95 A **True**   Viral hepatitis has little effect upon pregnancy,
      B **False** although occasionally fetal hepatitis may develop
      C **True**   and lead to stillbirth or neonatal death. If the
      D **True**   mother's nutritional status is poor it may
      E **True**   predispose her to acute hepatic necrosis, but in
                    general hepatitis is unaffected by the pregnancy.

3.96 A **False** *Trichomonas vaginalis* infestation causes local
      B **True**   pruritus vulvae. Syphilic rashes characteristically do
      C **True**   not itch.
      D **True**
      E **False**

3.97 Ulcerative colitis
A   has its greatest incidence in women of reproductive age
B   impairs fertility
C   usually becomes worse in pregnancy
D   increases the incidence of intrauterine growth retardation
E   does not usually increase the perinatal mortality rate

3.98 Severe heartburn in pregnancy
A   is more common in primigravidae
B   gets worse as pregnancy progresses
C   usually disappears within a few days of delivery
D   is caused by an increased secretion of gastric acid
E   is best treated by antacids and keeping the patient upright

3.99 On routine testing in the antenatal clinic the urine of a 32-week-pregnant woman shows the presence of protein. This is likely to be due to
A   urinary tract infection
B   pre-eclampsia
C   acute nephritis
D   polycystic disease of the kidney
E   contamination with vaginal discharge

3.100 Systemic lupus erythematosus in pregnancy
A   is very rare
B   leads to an increased risk of fetal cardiac anomalies
C   usually goes into remission
D   increases the risk of intrauterine fetal death
E   is treated with corticosteroids

3.101 In a pregnancy after renal transplantation the following are more likely to occur
A   spontaneous abortion
B   pre-eclampsia
C   intrauterine growth retardation
D   premature delivery
E   obstructed labour

3.102 In pregnancy, plasma concentration of phenytoin is affected by
A   absorption from the gastrointestinal tract at a faster rate than in non-pregnant patients
B   reduced protein binding
C   dilution in the increased plasma volume
D   increased hepatic hydroxylation
E   increased urine phenytoin concentration

(Answers overleaf)

3.97 A **True**   Ulcerative colitis is more common in women than
      B **False**   men, occurs mostly in the child bearing years and
      C **True**   does not impair fertility. The response of the
      D **False**   disease to pregnancy is variable, but 50% of those
      E **True**   with active disease will get worse. Ulcerative colitis
                     has no discernable effect upon pregnancy.

3.98 A **False**   Heartburn in pregnancy is due to reflux
      B **True**   oesophagitis and may be associated with hiatus
      C **True**   hernia. It is probably caused by a combination of
      D **False**   progesterone induced relaxation of gut muscle,
      E **True**   increased emptying time of the stomach and the
                     increasing uterine mass in the abdomen. It gets
                     worse as pregnancy progresses and is more
                     common in multigravidae.

3.99 A **True**   Most commonly protein found on routine testing is
      B **True**   a contaminant. If the protein is still present in a
      C **False**   midstream specimen it is most likely to be due to
      D **False**   urinary tract infection or pre-eclampsia. Acute
      E **True**   nephritis is very uncommon in pregnancy, as is
                     polycystic disease which generally appears in a
                     different age group.

3.100 A **False** SLE is an uncommon, but not rare condition, that
       B **True**   affects women of reproductive age. The effect of
       C **False** the disease on pregnancy is variable, but it
       D **True**   frequently gets worse, requiring treatment with
       E **True**   corticosteroids. If lupus anticoagulant is present the
                     intrauterine fetal death rate is increased. The
                     increase in fetal cardiac anomalies is related to
                     transplacental passage of maternal antibody.

3.101 A **False** Abortion is no more likely than in a normal
       B **True**   pregnancy. Approximately 30% of these women
       C **True**   develop pre-eclampsia, 20% intrauterine growth
       D **True**   retardation and about 50% are delivered early,
       E **False** usually electively. Although the transplanted kidney
                     is usually placed in the pelvis, obstructed labour is
                     not a consequence.

3.102 A **False** In pregnancy less phenytoin is absorbed from the
       B **True**   gut, more is hydroxylated in the liver and the
       C **True**   plasma concentration is further reduced by dilution.
       D **True**   On the other hand, protein binding is decreased,
       E **False** increasing free phenytoin levels, and renal
                     excretion is unchanged. Epileptics taking phenytoin
                     need their plasma drug levels measured frequently
                     to ensure that they are in the therapeutic range.

3.103   **The following are more likely to occur or get worse during pregnancy**
   A   carpal tunnel syndrome
   B   migraine
   C   Bell's palsy
   D   multiple sclerosis
   E   epilepsy

3.104   **Pemphigoid (herpes) gestationis**
   A   is pruritic
   B   is at its worst just before term
   C   recurs in subsequent pregnancies
   D   is vesicular
   E   is a contraindication to breast feeding

3.105   **In the United Kingdom HIV infection in pregnancy is a cause of**
   A   an increase in the congenital anomaly rate
   B   intrauterine growth retardation
   C   spontaneous premature labour
   D   fetal distress in labour
   E   premature rupture of the membranes

LABOUR

3.106   **The initiation of labour involves increased**
   A   fetal corticosteroid production
   B   placental oestradiol production
   C   placental progesterone production
   D   ovarian steroid hormone production
   E   uterine prostaglandin production

3.107   **Symptoms and signs of the onset of labour are**
   A   engagement of the fetal head
   B   uterine contractions
   C   dilatation of the cervix
   D   the show
   E   backache

3.108   **In labour, uterine contractions**
   A   originate in the lower segment
   B   are stronger in the upper than lower segment
   C   last longer in the upper than lower segment
   D   lead to temporary ischaemia in the myometrium
   E   are under voluntary control

(Answers overleaf)

3.103   A **True**   In carpal tunnel syndrome and Bell's palsy, nerves
        B **False**   pass through narrow bony canals. Oedema in
        C **True**   pregnancy causes pressure on the nerves to
        D **False**   increase. The effects are reversible. Migraine is
        E **True**   improved in pregnancy, as is multiple sclerosis
                        (which gets worse in the puerperium). The increase
                        in epileptic fits is mainly due to under-treatment in
                        pregnancy.

3.104   A **True**   Pemphigoid gestationis is an intensely pruritic
        B **False**   condition of pregnancy. Vesicular lesions enlarge
        C **True**   into bullae. There is usually remission for a few
        D **True**   weeks before term, but exacerbation after delivery.
        E **False**   Breast feeding may reduce the problem. Recurrence
                        in subsequent pregnancies is almost inevitable.

3.105   A **False**   There is still much uncertainty about the effects of
        B **False**   HIV positivity in pregnancy. Early concerns
        C **False**   regarding complications of pregnancy have largely
        D **False**   proved to be unfounded. Although many
        E **False**   complications of pregnancy are increased in these
                        women, this is generally not related to HIV status
                        but rather to lifestyle and social factors.

LABOUR

3.106   A **True**   The initiation of labour in the human is poorly
        B **True**   understood, but is likely to be the response to a
        C **False**   variety of factors. Fetal cortisol production
        D **False**   increases, suppressing placental progesterone and
        E **True**   increasing oestrogen production. The ovaries have
                        little if any effect as their steroid production is a
                        fraction of that from the placenta. The end point is
                        probably an increase in uterine prostaglandins
                        causing contractions.

3.107   A **False**   The timing of engagement of the presenting part is
        B **False**   only loosely related to the onset of labour. Uterine
        C **True**   contractions occur throughout pregnancy (and
        D **True**   reproductive life); it is painful, regular, frequent
        E **False**   contractions leading to dilatation of the cervix that
                        denote labour.

3.108   A **False**   Uterine contractions originate near the cornu and
        B **True**   spread throughout the uterus. They are stronger
        C **True**   and last longer in the upper segment. Compression
        D **True**   of the vessels during contractions leads to
        E **False**   temporary ischaemia, probably the cause of the
                        pain.

3.109 In the normal first stage of labour the fetal head

A   usually enters the pelvis in the pelvic antero-posterior diameter
B   rotates when it comes into contact with the pelvic floor
C   extends in the mid cavity
D   descends in an occipito-anterior position
E   is responsible for dilating the cervix

3.110 The normal second stage of labour

A   begins with full dilatation of the cervix
B   is accompanied by the strongest and most painful contractions of the whole labour
C   ends with delivery of the fetal head
D   A involves extension of the fetal head
E   involves external rotation of the fetal head to face laterally

3.111 Progress in labour is measured by

A   the frequency of uterine contractions
B   the force of uterine contractions
C   dilatation of the cervix
D   descent of the presenting part
E   the length of time since rupture of the membranes

3.112 In a normal primigravid labour

A   the rate of dilatation of the cervix is constant
B   the maximum rate of dilatation is approximately 1 cm per hour
C   the head engages in the first stage
D   the membranes should not be ruptured artificially before full dilatation
E   the duration is usually between eight and 12 hours

3.113 Pethidine can be used for analgesia in labour, but it

A   is not effective in one third of cases
B   causes nausea
C   causes neonatal respiratory depression if given within one of hour of delivery
D   depresses myometrial activity
E   must be given intravenously

(Answers overleaf)

3.109 A **False**   In normal labour the head enters the pelvis in the
       B **True**   wider, transverse diameter and rotates in contact
       C **False**   with the pelvic floor to the occipito-anterior position
       D **True**   which presents the smallest diameter. The head is
       E **False**   flexed until it emerges through the pelvic outlet.
                       Dilatation is a function of uterine activity, not fetal
                       pressure.

3.110 A **True**   The second stage of labour begins at full cervical
       B **False**   dilatation and ends with delivery of the fetus.
       C **False**   Contractions are not as painful as in the late first
       D **True**   stage. At delivery the fetal head extends and the
       E **True**   perineum sweeps across the face. The shoulders
                       enter the pelvis in the transverse diameter and
                       rotate to the antero-posterior diameter, causing the
                       head to turn to face the thigh.

3.111 A **False**   Progress is measured by dilatation of the cervix and
       B **False**   descent of the presenting part. It may be
       C **True**   satisfactory in the absence of strong, frequent
       D **True**   contractions, or may be unsatisfactory even when
       E **False**   the contractions appear adequate. Labours vary in
                       length and progress is not necessarily related to the
                       time taken.

3.112 A **False**   Cervical dilatation is slow at first, but accelerates to
       B **True**   approximately 1 cm per hour once the cervix is
       C **False**   dilated to approximately 3 cm. Engagement should
       D **False**   take place before labour begins. ARM should be
       E **True**   performed as soon as it is safe to do so in order to
                       reveal any meconium in the liquor and to enable
                       internal continuous fetal heart rate monitoring to be
                       employed if necessary.

3.113 A **True**   Pethidine is still widely used as an analgesic in
       B **True**   labour, despite the associated nausea and its
       C **False**   failure, partial or total, to control the pain in 30–40%
       D **False**   of women. It has no effect on myometrial activity.
       E **False**   Despite the widely held belief that pethidine given
                       shortly (1–2 hours) before delivery depresses
                       respiration in the neonate, it is actually the
                       pethidine given approximately four hours or more
                       before delivery that has this effect.

3.114 Contraindications to the use of epidural anaesthesia in labour include

A   coagulopathies
B   prolonged labour
C   breech delivery
D   multiple pregnancy
E   caesarean section

3.115 Epid mural anaesthesia in labour

A   produces total pain relief
B   decreases the woman's ability to push the fetus out
C   depresses neonatal respiration
D   relaxes the levator ani muscles
E   interferes with the internal rotation of the fetal head

3.116 Premature labour

A   is effectively stopped with intravenous ritodrine
B   is stopped by administering corticosteroids
C   only occurs before 32 weeks gestation
D   should be managed by caesarean section
E   is more frequently complicated by a breech presentation than labour at term

3.117 Complications of induction of labour include

A   postpartum haemorrhage
B   failure to establish labour
C   prematurity
D   maternal hypertension
E   intrauterine sepsis

3.118 The Bishop score includes the

A   gestational age
B   engagement of the presenting part
C   station of the presenting part
D   effacement of the cervix
E   dilatation of the cervix

3.119 Agents effective in ripening the unfavourable cervix before term include

A   laminaria tents
B   extra-amniotic prostaglandin E_2
C   intravenous Syntocinon
D   intravaginal prostaglandins
E   oral Syntocinon

(Answers overleaf)

3.114 A **True**   Epidural anaesthesia is effective in abolishing the
      B **False**   pain of contractions in most patients. Absolute
      C **False**   contraindications are few, but include coagulopathy,
      D **False**   because of the risk of bleeding into the epidural
      E **False**   space. Epidural anaesthesia is entirely appropriate,
                    and indeed helpful, in the other cases listed.

3.115 A **True**   Epidurals are effective analgesics which, unlike
      B **False**   opiates, do not depress neonatal respiration. The
      C **False**   woman is quite capable of pushing, uterine
      D **True**   contractions and abdominal wall muscles are
      E **True**   unaffected, but because the levators relax the fetal
                    head frequently fails to rotate when it reaches the
                    pelvic floor, leading to an increased rotational
                    forceps rate.

3.116 A **False**   Premature labour is any labour occurring before 37
      B **False**   weeks gestation. Although labour may be slowed
      C **False**   by ritodrine it is not stopped. Steroids are
      D **False**   frequently given to hasten lung maturity. Breech
      E **True**   presentation is more common the more premature
                    the labour, but those cases presenting by the head
                    can usually be delivered vaginally.

3.117 A **False**   The complications of induction of labour are
      B **True**   delivery of a premature infant (deliberately or
      C **True**   because of mistaken dates), introduction of
      D **False**   infection and the failure of labour to begin.
      E **True**

3.118 A **False**   The Bishop score is a measure of the favourability
      B **False**   of the cervix for induction of labour. It includes
      C **True**   dilatation, position, consistency and effacement of
      D **True**   the cervix and the station of the presenting part.
      E **True**   High scores are more favourable.

3.119 A **True**   Syntocinon is not effective in ripening the
      B **True**   unfavourable cervix regardless of the route of
      C **False**   administration. Local application of prostaglandins
      D **True**   is effective and relatively safe. Laminaria tents swell
      E **False**   in the cervix and cause ripening, but are associated
                    with an unacceptable level of infection.

3.120 **In labour, fetal heart rate patterns that are indications for fetal blood sampling include**
- A a persistent rate of 175 bpm
- B accelerations with contractions
- C late decelerations
- D a persistent rate of 125 bpm
- E a baseline variability of 10 bpm

3.121 **Fetal blood sampling**
- A is not possible with a fetus presenting by the breech
- B leads to clinically significant fetal haemorrhage in 5% of cases
- C may lead to transient fetal bradycardia
- D is rarely followed by formation of a scalp abscess
- E is used to obtain fetal capillary blood

3.122 **Cord prolapse**
- A should always be treated by immediate caesarean section
- B is commonly associated with a malpresentation
- C usually follows artificial rupture of the membranes
- D is frequently associated with multiple pregnancy
- E is frequently associated with prematurity

3.123 **Delay in labour is associated with**
- A previous caesarean section
- B an android pelvis
- C oligohydramnios
- D engagement of the fetal head in the transverse position
- E occipito-posterior position

3.124 **A fetus with a face presentation in labour**
- A is found in approximately 1 in 500 deliveries
- B will usually only deliver if the position is mento-anterior
- C should be delivered by caesarean section
- D has a major congenital abnormality in most cases
- E will usually deliver vaginally

3.125 **During the first stage of labour**
- A early decelerations are frequently associated with fetal acidosis
- B late decelerations are always associated with significant fetal acidosis
- C there is a progressive fall in the pH of fetal blood
- D maternal pyrexia may cause fetal tachycardia
- E variable decelerations may be due to cord compression

(Answers overleaf)

3.120 A **True**   Fetal blood sampling should be performed when
       B **False**   meconium is seen or when the fetal heart rate is
       C **True**   abnormal. A normal fetal heart rate pattern has a
       D **False**   baseline between 120 and 160 bpm, with a baseline
       E **False**   variability of approximately 10 bpm and
                      accelerations with contractions.

3.121 A **False**   Fetal capillary blood may be taken from the scalp or
       B **False**   buttock. Significant unwanted haemorrhage occurs
       C **True**   in only 0.3% and scalp infection in 0.3% of cases.
       D **True**   Transient fetal bradycardia may be due to pressure
       E **True**   of the amnioscope on the fetal head.

3.122 A **False**   Cord prolapse is more frequent when the
       B **True**   presenting part does not fit snugly into the pelvis
       C **False**   such as with malpresentations, prematurity, or
       D **True**   multiple pregnancy. Caesarean section is often not
       E **True**   necessary, as in the second stage of labour or with
                      a dead fetus. It is more common after spontaneous
                      than artificial rupture of the membranes.

3.123 A **False**   Delay in labour is most frequently due to
       B **True**   inadequate contractions or too large a presenting
       C **False**   part. In an android pelvis the shape of the pelvis
       D **False**   leads to disproportion. In an occipito-posterior
       E **True**   position a larger diameter of the fetal head
                      presents, slowing labour. The fetal head engages in
                      the transverse position normally.

3.124 A **True**   As a mento-anterior presentation descends
       B **True**   extension takes place, holding the fetus in a face
       C **False**   presentation. A mento-posterior presentation will
       D **False**   flex as it descends, turning into a brow and
       E **True**   presenting a larger diameter. Most cases of face
                      presentation are entirely normal and deliver
                      vaginally with a minimum of problems.

3.125 A **False**   Early fetal heart rate decelerations, with
       B **False**   contractions, are said to be due to pressure on the
       C **True**   fetal head and are not associated with fetal distress.
       D **True**   Late decelerations may indicate fetal distress, but
       E **True**   should lead to fetal blood sampling as the fetus is
                      frequently not acidotic. Variable decelerations are
                      said to be due to cord compression. Maternal
                      pyrexia and tachycardia are often associated with
                      fetal tachycardia.

3.126 Brow presentation
A is usually recognised in the second stage of labour
B leads to prolonged labour
C is usually an indication to perform caesarean section
D is treated by flexion to a vertex presentation
E can sometimes be delivered with forceps

3.127 A classical caesarean section
A should be considered in cases of transverse lie
B is performed when large fibroids occupy the lower segment of the uterus
C is performed in most cases of placenta praevia
D is performed through a transverse incision in the upper segment of the uterus
E scar is liable to rupture after 30 weeks gestation

3.128 Caesarean section should be performed on all patients
A who have had two or more previous caesarean sections
B with grade 3 placenta praevia
C who have had a previous caesarean section for fetal distress
D with cord prolapse
E who have diabetes mellitus

3.129 Rotational (Kielland's) forceps
A can be used to correct asynclitism
B are used when the head is not engaged
C are used to correct deep transverse arrest
D should not be used with pudendal block anaesthesia alone
E cause a small fall in fetal blood pH

3.130 Indications for immediate delivery using forceps include
A delay late in the first stage of labour
B delay in the second stage of labour
C fetal heart rate decelerations with contractions in the second stage of labour
D severe fetal distress late in the first stage of labour
E persistent fetal bradycardia in the second stage of labour

(Answers overleaf)

3.126   A   **False**   In a brow presentation the mento-vertical diameter
        B   **True**   presents. It is usually recognised in the first stage
        C   **True**   of labour when investigating the cause of
        D   **False**   prolonged labour. Occasionally recognition occurs
        E   **True**   late in the second stage, and if the pelvis is
                        particularly capacious it may be possible to deliver
                        the fetus by extension to a face presentation or
                        with forceps.

3.127   A   **True**   Classical section scars rupture in the last 10 weeks
        B   **True**   of pregnancy rather than in labour and are very
        C   **False**   dangerous. It should only be performed rarely, such
        D   **False**   as in cases of transverse lie with the limbs
        E   **True**   uppermost or fibroids in the lower segment. A
                        longitudinal midline incision is made in the upper
                        segment.

3.128   A   **True**   Repeat caesarean section depends upon the cause
        B   **True**   for the original section. If it was disproportion it
        C   **False**   should be repeated, but if it was fetal distress the
        D   **False**   patient may labour normally. If she has had more
        E   **False**   than one caesarean section she should not be
                        allowed to labour again. With grade 3 placenta
                        praevia safe vaginal delivery is impossible. Cord
                        prolapse in the second stage calls for delivery with
                        forceps. Although more than 60% of diabetics have
                        caesarean sections, it is not mandatory.

3.129   A   **True**   The sliding lock in Kielland's forceps is used to
        B   **False**   correct asynclitism. They are used to turn the fetal
        C   **True**   head from the transverse or occipito-posterior
        D   **True**   position to the occipito-anterior position, but must
        E   **True**   only be used if the head is deeply engaged. This is
                        a painful procedure requiring epidural, spinal, or
                        general anaesthesia. A small fall in fetal pH occurs.

3.130   A   **False**   Forceps should only be used to deliver a fetus in
        B   **True**   the second stage of labour, never in the first stage
        C   **False**   because of causing damage to maternal structures
        D   **False**   and, potentially the fetus. If delivery needs to be
        E   **True**   expedited in the first stage caesarean section is
                        necessary. Heart rate decelerations with
                        contractions in the second stage of labour are
                        physiological.

3.131 When delivering the second twin vaginally

A   Syntocinon is contraindicated
B   malpresentations are common
C   epidural anaesthesia is an advantage
D   the membranes must be allowed to rupture
spontaneously
E   internal podalic version may occasionally be necessary

3.132 The Ventouse is used to deliver the fetus

A   when the head is in the occipito-anterior position
B   when the head is in the occipito-posterior position
C   when the head is in the transverse position
D   presenting by the face
E   presenting by the brow

3.133 When delivering a fetus presenting by the breech

A   Syntocinon should not be used
B   caesarean section is the preferred route with a footling
breech
C   traction on the trunk leads to extension of the arms
D   Lovsetts manoeuvre is used to deliver the head
E   meconium can be ignored

3.134 The Apgar score

A   is a measure of fetal well-being
B   relates well to umbilical vein pH
C   includes a score for fetal heart rate
D   includes a score for neonatal respiratory function
E   is measured 15 minutes after delivery

(Answers overleaf)

3.131 A **False**   The second twin is at greater risk than the first.
       B **True**   Malpresentations are common and must be
       C **True**   corrected by external version, although
       D **False**   occasionally, immediately after rupture of the
       E **True**   membranes, it may be necessary to perform
                      internal podalic version to correct a transverse lie.
                      Once the lie is longitudinal the membranes should
                      be ruptured artificially and the presenting part
                      allowed to descend into the pelvis.

3.132 A **True**   The Ventouse can be used instead of forceps to
       B **True**   deliver term babies with any position of the fetal
       C **True**   head, but only when the presentation is vertex or
       D **False**   occipito-posterior (deflexed but not to a brow or
       E **False**   face).

3.133 A **False**   Although any type of breech can be delivered
       B **True**   vaginally the success rate is much greater with the
       C **True**   extended breech and many obstetricians would
       D **False**   prefer to perform caesarean section on a flexed and
       E **False**   particularly a footling breech. Although Syntocinon
                      is to be avoided whenever possible during labour
                      and certainly not used to overcome secondary
                      arrest (which usually denotes disproportion) there
                      is no absolute contraindication to its use when it is
                      suspected that uterine inertia is the cause of delay.
                      Although the passage of meconium during the
                      breech delivery is common and is often of no
                      significance it must always be investigated as it
                      may denote fetal distress. During the delivery of the
                      fetus traction on the trunk leads to extension of the
                      arms which can be corrected using Lovsetts
                      manoeuvre. The head is usually delivered with
                      forceps.

3.134 A **True**   The Apgar score is taken at 1, 5 and 10 minutes
       B **False**   after delivery as a measure of neonatal well-being.
       C **True**   Unfortunately it does not relate well to fetal pH
       D **True**   except at the extremes. It is a measure of neonatal
       E **False**   heart rate, respiration, colour, tone and response to
                      stimulus.

3.135 The third stage of labour
  A   begins with separation of the placenta
  B   ends with delivery of the placenta
  C   is associated with the return of the uterus to its pre-
      pregnant size
  D   is accompanied by an average blood loss of 600 ml
  E   is normally actively managed in the UK

**3.136 The following changes take place in the uterus in the third
stage of labour**
  A   uterine contractions are less frequent than in the second
      stage of labour
  B   the intrauterine pressure during contractions is less than
      in the second stage of labour
  C   myometrial fibres retract
  D   the decidual surface area is reduced
  E   the upper segment is more affected than the lower
      segment

**3.137 In the third stage of labour, signs of separation of the
placenta are**
  A   vaginal bleeding
  B   an increase in uterine mobility
  C   widening of the uterine body
  D   lengthening of the umbilical cord
  E   the patient experiences pain

3.138 In the active management of the third stage of labour
  A   the uterus must be contracted
  B   fundal pressure is applied
  C   the placenta is delivered by pulling on the cord as soon
      as the baby has been delivered
  D   the patient is usually given ergometrine intramuscularly
  E   intravenous Syntocinon is effective

3.139 In the third stage of labour, ergometrine
  A   given intravenously acts immediately
  B   is given in a dose of 50 mg
  C   is an emetic
  D   may cause hypertension
  E   is usually given in combination with Syntocinon

(Answers overleaf)

3.135   A **False**   The third stage of labour begins after delivery of
        B **True**   the fetus and ends with delivery of the placenta.
        C **False**   Placental separation is an event during the third
        D **False**   stage. The average blood loss is 200–400 ml and
        E **True**   although the uterus becomes smaller, complete
                        involution will usually take several weeks. Active
                        management of the third stage with oxytocics is the
                        usual practice in order to reduce the incidence of
                        postpartum haemorrhage.

3.136   A **False**   In the third stage of labour the myometrial fibres
        B **False**   contract and retract. The upper segment is reduced
        C **True**   in size and the area of the decidual surface is
        D **True**   reduced. The contractions are the equal of those
        E **True**   seen in late first and the second stage of labour in
                        terms of frequency and pressure generated.

3.137   A **True**   Signs of placental separation include vaginal
        B **True**   bleeding, narrowing of the uterine body so that the
        C **False**   uterus becomes more globular and mobile and
        D **True**   lengthening of the cord. Separation itself is not
        E **False**   painful.

3.138   A **True**   In the active management of the third stage an
        B **False**   oxytocic such as intravenous Syntocinon,
        C **False**   intramuscular Syntometrine or, rarely nowadays,
        D **False**   intravenous ergometrine is given to the mother.
        E **True**   The placenta is delivered by controlled cord traction
                        after placental separation and only when the uterus
                        is contracted. The combination of cord traction
                        before placental separation and a relaxed uterus
                        may lead to uterine inversion, perhaps even more
                        likely if accompanied by fundal pressure, which is
                        usually ineffective anyway.

3.139   A **True**   Ergometrine is the most effective agent in causing
        B **False**   tonic uterine contraction, acting immediately when
        C **True**   given intravenously (6–7 min intramuscularly). A
        D **True**   dose of 0.5 mg is used. Because of the side-effects
        E **True**   of vomiting and transient hypertension,
                        ergometrine is only given intravenously to control
                        severe haemorrhage from atonic uterus, or
                        intramuscularly in combination with 5 units of
                        Syntocinon (Syntometrine), an agent that combines
                        the relatively rapid effect of Syntocinon with the
                        long lasting effect of intramuscular ergometrine. In
                        many cases intravenous Syntocinon is preferred in
                        the third stage of labour.

3.140 After delivery the following must always be inspected
A the placenta
B the umbilical cord
C the lower vagina
D the cervix
E the lower uterine segment (digitally)

3.141 Primary postpartum haemorrhage
A can occur at any time in the first week after delivery
B frequently occurs in association with the third stage of labour
C is usually due to a coagulation failure
D is due to complete failure of separation of the placenta
E is commonly due to uterine inertia

3.142 Primary postpartum haemorrhage is associated with
A placenta praevia
B polyhydramnios
C multiple pregnancy
D forceps delivery
E prolonged labour

3.143 Primary postpartum haemorrhage occurs more commonly
A in primigravidae
B when there is a history of a previous postpartum haemorrhage
C when fibroids are present in the uterus
D in premature labour
E after placental abruption

(Answers overleaf)

3.140 A **True** Postpartum haemorrhage is frequently due to
       B **True** retained parts of the placenta, and the placenta
       C **True** should always be inspected to ensure that it is
       D **False** complete. The vessels in the cord need to be
       E **False** counted. The absence of one of the arteries is
                    associated with fetal anomaly in 25% of cases. The
                    perineum and lower vagina are inspected for tears,
                    but unless there is heavy bleeding it is not
                    necessary, and is uncomfortable for the patient, to
                    inspect the upper vagina or cervix. Even when the
                    patient has had a previous caesarean section it is
                    not necessary to palpate the lower segment of the
                    uterus.

3.141 A **False** Primary postpartum haemorrhage occurs in the first
       B **True** 24 hours after delivery. It is most common in the
       C **False** first 2–3 hours, often during the third stage of
       D **False** labour. Causes are uterine atony, trauma to the
       E **True** genital tract and, much less commonly, coagulation
                    failure. Complete failure of separation of the
                    placenta does not lead to bleeding, it is partial
                    separation, or separation without expulsion, both of
                    which cause uterine atony, which lead to
                    postpartum haemorrhage.

3.142 A **True** Over-distension of the uterus or prolonged labour
       B **True** leads to a failure of adequate myometrial
       C **True** contraction in the third stage. Operative delivery
       D **True** increases the likelihood of bleeding from trauma to
       E **True** the genital tract. The lower segment of the uterus,
                    the site of the placental bed in placenta praevia,
                    contracts less well than the upper segment.

3.143 A **False** Postpartum haemorrhage is more common in
       B **True** grand multipara who have a larger proportion of
       C **True** fibrous to muscular tissue in the uterus. Postpartum
       D **False** haemorrhage is a recurrent factor from one
       E **True** pregnancy to another. Multiple fibroids may
                    interfere with uterine contraction. After placental
                    abruption there may be hypofibrinogenaemia and a
                    coagulation problem; in addition, raised fibrin
                    degradation product concentrations relax the uterus.

3.144 Manual removal of the placenta
  A is performed using a pudendal block as analgesia
  B has been superseded by the use of the suction curette
  C should only be performed when the uterus is contracted
  D should be performed if the fetal membranes are ragged
  E is an indication for giving prophylactic antibiotics

3.145 Uterine rupture in labour
  A most commonly occurs after classical caesarean section
  B is common after tubal reanastomosis
  C is commoner in primigravidae
  D is a complication of internal podalic version
  E is more common if the uterus has previously been
     perforated at termination of pregnancy

3.146 Signs of uterine rupture in labour include
  A heavy vaginal bleeding
  B strong uterine contractions
  C fetal death
  D maternal tachycardia
  E constant abdominal pain

3.147 Paravaginal haematomas
  A always follow forceps delivery
  B usually resolve spontaneously
  C often require surgical intervention
  D frequently have no identifiable source
  E are a cause of collapse postpartum

3.148 Morbid adherence of the placenta
  A is associated with placenta praevia
  B should be managed by removal of as much of the
     placenta as is possible
  C is associated with a previous caesarean section
  D necessitates hysterectomy
  E commonly involves invasion through to the serosal coat
     of the uterus

(Answers overleaf)

3.144 A **False**   Manual removal of the placenta is painful and
      B **False**   requires epidural, spinal or general anaesthesia.
      C **False**   Use of a curette is dangerous, uterine perforation is
      D **False**   very likely. The uterus is relaxed, otherwise you
      E **True**   cannot get a hand inside. Ragged membranes are
                    frequently seen and are usually of no consequence.
                    Inevitably the infection risk is increased when
                    manual removal of the placenta is performed.

3.145 A **False**   Uterine rupture after classical caesarean section
      B **False**   often occurs in late pregnancy; classical caesarean
      C **False**   section is now rarely seen anyway. Tubal
      D **True**   reimplantation leads to a weakness in the uterine
      E **True**   wall, as does previous uterine perforation, but not
                    tubal reanastomosis. Rupture virtually always
                    occurs in multigravidae. Internal podalic version is
                    now rarely performed, partly because of the risk of
                    uterine rupture.

3.146 A **False**   Uterine rupture is associated with an intrapartum
      B **False**   vaginal blood loss, usually relatively slight, a
      C **True**   cessation of uterine contractions, constant lower
      D **True**   abdominal pain, maternal shock and fetal death.
      E **True**

3.147 A **False**   Paravaginal haematomas may follow normal or
      B **False**   forceps deliveries and can become very large very
      C **True**   quickly. They are managed surgically, unlike broad
      D **True**   ligament haematomas that usually resolve
      E **True**   spontaneously. Usually no single bleeding point is
                    found, treatment being by evacuation of the clot
                    and drainage.

3.148 A **True**   Cases of morbid adherence of the placenta are
      B **False**   divided into three grades of increasing severity and
      C **True**   decreasing frequency, accreta, increta and finally
      D **False**   the rare percreta when the chorionic villi penetrate
      E **False**   through the serosal coat of the uterus. Placenta
                    accreta, the commonest grade, is associated with
                    placenta praevia, the presence of a previous
                    caesarean section scar or, more frequently, both of
                    these together. If the placenta has not separated at
                    all it should be left in place and managed
                    conservatively. If it has partly separated, bleeding is
                    such that hysterectomy is almost inevitable.

3.149 Uterine inversion

    A   only occurs with a relaxed uterus

    B   is usually caused by applying fundal pressure

    C   is managed by immediate removal of the placenta before replacing the uterus

    D   is managed by increasing the hydrostatic pressure in the vagina

    E   requires hysterectomy

3.150 During an assisted breech delivery

    A   analgesia may be effected by pudendal nerve block

    B   epidural anaesthesia is contraindicated

    C   an episiotomy should be performed when the fetal anus appears at the vulva

    D   the second stage should not last for more than one hour

    E   forceps are used to deliver the after-coming head

THE PUERPERIUM

3.151 In the puerperium

    A   the uterine fundus is usually palpable at just below the umbilicus 10 days following delivery

    B   by six weeks the uterus has returned to a non-pregnant size

    C   lochia is usually red for 10 days

    D   lochia usually continues for about six weeks

    E   in a non-breast feeding mother menstruation usually commences about six weeks after delivery

3.152 Breast development in pregnancy is characterised by

    A   an increase in vascularity

    B   the secretion of colostrum by Montgomery's tubercles

    C   oedema formation

    D   increased pigmentation of the areola

    E   duct development

(Answers overleaf)

3.149 A **True**   Inversion of the uterus is a rare complication of the
       B **False**   third stage of labour. It is caused by traction on the
       C **False**   cord before separation of a fundally placed placenta
       D **True**   when the uterus is relaxed. If the placenta is still in
       E **False**   place when the inversion is diagnosed it is left
                      alone to avoid provoking bleeding. Unless the
                      uterus can be replaced immediately the best
                      technique to use is O'Sullivan's which involves
                      running warm saline into the vagina, increasing the
                      hydrostatic pressure and gently forcing the uterus
                      back in place.

3.150 A **True**   Analgesia may be effected by pudendal block,
       B **False**   although because of the manipulations involved,
       C **True**   epidural anaesthesia is often helpful. An episiotomy
       D **True**   should not be performed too early as heavy
       E **True**   bleeding may occur, but once the fetal trunk is
                      delivered it is difficult to perform. If the second
                      stage of labour lasts for more than one hour then it
                      is likely that there is some disproportion and
                      caesarean section is a better option. Forceps are
                      frequently used to deliver the after-coming head
                      and are probably the safest technique.

THE PUERPERIUM

3.151 A **False**   The uterine fundus is usually palpable just below
       B **True**   the umbilicus immediately after delivery. After
       C **False**   about 10 days it is no longer palpable abdominally,
       D **False**   by six weeks it has returned to a non-pregnant size.
       E **True**   Lochia consists of red and white blood cells,
                      bacteria and decidua. In the first few days it is
                      mainly blood but becomes paler by the seventh
                      day. It usually ceases at about four weeks following
                      delivery. In women who are not breast feeding,
                      menstruation usually commences about six weeks
                      after delivery.

3.152 A **True**   During pregnancy, under the influence of
       B **False**   oestrogens and progesterone, there is increased
       C **False**   growth in the breast of ducts, alveoli and lobules.
       D **True**   There is increased vascularity, but fat, connective
       E **True**   tissue and oedema relatively decrease. The areola
                      becomes pigmented. Montgomery's tubercles are
                      sebaceous glands.

3.153 **Breast feeding is more likely to succeed if**
   A   the nipples are everted
   B   initial suckling is delayed until the mother has rested after delivery
   C   oral oestrogens are administered
   D   baby and mother share the same room
   E   supplementary cow's milk feeds are given

3.154 **Human breast milk contains**
   A   less protein than cow's milk
   B   less iron than cow's milk
   C   immunoglobulins which protect the infant from gastroenteritis
   D   alcohol if the mother drinks alcohol herself
   E   a constant balance of constituents

3.155 **During lactation**
   A   prolactin causes the myoepithelial cells of the breast to contract
   B   ovulation is often delayed
   C   prolactin secretion is stimulated by suckling
   D   the administration of a progestogen will suppress milk production
   E   oxytocin secretion is stimulated by suckling

3.156 **The following drugs are safe to use in breast feeding mothers**
   A   labetalol
   B   warfarin
   C   carbimazole
   D   insulin
   E   rifampicin

3.157 **Ergometrine**
   A   is an antiemetic
   B   should be given with caution to patients with hypertension
   C   acts immediately when given intramuscularly
   D   causes the uterus to contract rhythmically
   E   is more effective in causing uterine contractions in the third than the first trimester

(Answers overleaf)

3.153 A **True**   Successful breast feeding depends upon the
      B **False**   enthusiasm of the mother as well as
      C **False**   encouragement and education from her attendants.
      D **True**   The baby should be suckled as soon after delivery
      E **False**   as possible, initially for 2–3 minutes on each side,
                    and thereafter fed on demand. Supplementary
                    cow's milk feed should be kept to a minimum. Oral
                    oestrogens are used to suppress lactation.

3.154 A **False**   The composition of breast milk varies throughout
      B **True**   feed, the fat concentration rising towards the end.
      C **True**   Furthermore the composition may differ between
      D **True**   two feeds on the same day, and milk of the early
      E **False**   puerperium differs from that of established
                    lactation. It is a better source of protein than cow's
                    milk but contains relatively less iron. The
                    immunoglobulins present are one of several factors
                    increasing the resistance of the baby to
                    gastroenteritis. Many drugs including alcohol are
                    transmitted into breast milk in significant quantities.

3.155 A **False**   Oxytocin and prolactin secretion are stimulated by
      B **True**   suckling. The prolactin promotes milk synthesis
      C **True**   while the oxytocin causes milk ejection. Oestrogens
      D **False**   block the action of prolactin and suppress lactation,
      E **True**   progestogens have no effect. Ovulation is delayed
                    but not reliably, and lactation is not to be
                    recommended as an effective contraceptive
                    measure.

3.156 A **True**   Labetalol does not enter breast milk in significant
      B **True**   amounts, nor does insulin. Warfarin passes into
      C **False**   breast milk, but except in vitamin K deficiency
      D **True**   appears to be safe. Rifampicin also passes into
      E **True**   breast milk, but does not harm the infant.
                    Carbimazole causes neonatal hypothyroidism or
                    goitre.

3.157 A **False**   Ergometrine causes both gut and vascular smooth
      B **True**   muscle to contract. It is therefore emetic and may
      C **False**   make hypertension worse or precipitate heart
      D **False**   failure in susceptible patients. In the uterus it is
      E **True**   more effective after oestrogen priming and causes
                    a tonic contraction, immediately after intravenous
                    injection, but about seven minutes after an
                    intramuscular injection.

3.158 Uterine inversion
- A   may lead to Sheehan's syndrome
- B   usually causes heavy vaginal bleeding
- C   can be managed by O'Sullivan's technique
- D   frequently requires hysterectomy
- E   will not occur if the uterus is contracted

3.159 Secondary postpartum haemorrhage
- A   is defined as loss of more than 500 ml from the genital tract between 24 hours and six weeks after delivery
- B   is usually due to retained products of conception
- C   is frequently associated with uterine infection
- D   commonly requires a blood transfusion
- E   may require a total abdominal hysterectomy if severe

3.160 In a woman with a secondary postpartum haemorrhage two weeks following delivery
- A   the cervix is commonly open
- B   an ultrasound scan is often helpful
- C   oral ergometrine should be administered
- D   there is a significant risk of uterine perforation if an evacuation of the uterus is necessary
- E   if the woman has a high temperature and a very tender uterus immediate evacuation of the uterus is the correct management

3.161 In the absence of an obvious vaginal haemorrhage postpartum collapse may be due to
- A   a paravaginal haematoma
- B   a ruptured uterus
- C   amniotic fluid embolism
- D   eclampsia
- E   uterine inversion

(Answers overleaf)

3.158 A **True**   Partial or total uterine inversion will only occur
       B **False**   when the uterus is relaxed. Heavy bleeding may
       C **True**   occur, but this is unusual, although shock may be
       D **False**   profound enough to cause Sheehan's syndrome.
       E **True**   Treatment is by replacing the uterus either directly
                      or by O'Sullivan's technique using hydrostatic
                      pressure.

3.159 A **False**   The definition of secondary postpartum
       B **True**   haemorrhage is significant blood loss from the
       C **True**   genital tract between 24 hours and six weeks
       D **False**   following delivery. The amount of blood loss is not
       E **True**   specified. It is often due to retained products of
                      conception, frequently associated with pelvic
                      infection and failure of the placental bed to
                      involute. Only one in 10 cases are severe enough to
                      warrant a blood transfusion, but occasionally the
                      bleeding can be catastrophic and the woman may
                      require a total abdominal hysterectomy.

3.160 A **True**   There is usually sub-involution of the uterus and
       B **True**   the cervix is commonly open. An ultrasound scan
       C **False**   can help to confirm a diagnosis of retained
       D **True**   products of conception. The usual problem is
       E **False**   infection often with retained products of conception
                      and oral ergometrine is of little value. The uterus is
                      soft and frequently infected and there is a
                      significant risk of uterine perforation at evacuation
                      of the uterus. If a woman has a high temperature
                      and a very tender uterus it is much better to treat
                      the woman with intravenous antibiotics for at least
                      24 hours prior to evacuation of retained products.

3.161 A **True**   A paravaginal haematoma may contain litres of
       B **True**   blood and a ruptured uterus may lead to massive
       C **True**   intraperitoneal haemorrhage. Both can cause
       D **True**   collapse with hypovolaemic shock. Amniotic fluid
       E **True**   embolism and eclampsia cause coagulopathies and
                      cerebral haemorrhages. With uterine inversion the
                      shock produced is out of all proportion to the blood
                      loss.

3.162 **Puerperal pyrexia**

A is a temperature of 38°C on any occasion in the first six weeks following delivery or miscarriage
B is commonly due to deep venous thrombosis
C may be due to acute mastitis
D may be caused by an upper respiratory tract infection
E is commonly due to an infected episiotomy site

3.163 **The management of a woman with a puerperal pyrexia should include**

A checking a full blood count
B taking a midstream urine specimen
C taking a high vaginal swab for culture and sensitivity
D suppression of lactation
E treatment with broad spectrum antibiotics

3.164 **Predisposing factors in the development of puerperal infection are**

A haemorrhage
B trauma to the genital tract
C prolonged labour
D retained placenta
E anaemia

3.165 **Deep venous thrombosis in the puerperium**

A is very common and can generally be treated with analgesics and bed rest
B is a contraindication to the progestogen only pill for contraception
C is more common in women over the age of 35 years
D is a contraindication to suppression of lactation with stilboestrol
E should always be treated with anticoagulants

3.166 **In the puerperium deep venous thrombosis should be treated**

A by embolectomy
B with heparin
C by resting the patient in bed
D with analgesics
E with vigorous leg exercises

(Answers overleaf)

3.162 A **False** A puerperal pyrexia is defined as a temperature of
      B **False** 38°C on any occasion on the first 14 days following
      C **True**   delivery or miscarriage. It can be caused by urinary
      D **True**   tract infection, genital tract infection, breast
      E **False** infection, or coincidental infection, e.g. upper
                   respiratory tract infection. It is only rarely due to
                   deep venous thrombosis. Infected episiotomy sites
                   tend to cause a localised infection and only rarely
                   produce a generalised infection.

3.163 A **True**   It is important to take a full history and to examine
      B **True**   the patient. Investigations should include a full
      C **True**   blood count, a midstream urine specimen and a
      D **False** high vaginal swab. Suppression of lactation is only
      E **True**   necessary if there is a severe breast infection.
                   Treatment once the relevant investigations have
                   been performed should be prompt and include
                   broad spectrum antibiotics.

3.164 A **True**   Retained products provide a good medium for the
      B **True**   growth of infection. Removal of the placenta and
      C **True**   any other form of operative intervention
      D **True**   traumatises the maternal tissues and may introduce
      E **True**   infection. The infection rate is related to the time
                   spent in labour and to the general state of the
                   patient.

3.165 A **False** Deep venous thrombosis in the puerperium is more
      B **False** common with advancing maternal age and should
      C **True**   always be treated with anticoagulants. It is not
      D **True**   made worse by progestogens but is by oestrogens
      E **True**   which should be avoided.

3.166 A **False** Deep venous thrombosis in the puerperium is
      B **True**   treated with anticoagulants, heparin initially and
      C **True**   then warfarin, analgesia and bed rest. Vigorous
      D **True**   exercise will be painful and may increase the risk of
      E **False** embolisation.

3.167 The following are risk factors for deep venous thrombosis in the puerperium

A   postpartum sterilisation
B   suppression of lactation with oestrogens
C   an epidural in labour
D   intravenous Syntocinon in labour
E   forceps delivery

3.168 Superficial thrombophlebitis in the puerperium

A   occurs in about 5% of pregnancies
B   should be treated by anticoagulation
C   predisposes to pulmonary embolism
D   may cause a puerperal pyrexia
E   should be treated with antibiotics

3.169 In the puerperium pulmonary embolism

A   is the usual consequence of deep venous thrombosis
B   is a major cause of maternal death
C   should be treated by anticoagulating the patient
D   may present with sudden collapse of the patient
E   is usually preceded by signs and symptoms of a deep vein thrombosis

3.170 The 'maternity blues'

A   occur in about 10% of patients following delivery
B   usually require treatment with mild anxiolytics
C   are less likely in breast feeding mothers
D   usually occur within 48 hours of delivery
E   are almost certainly due to the endocrine changes of the puerperium

(Answers overleaf)

3.167   A   **True**   The risk of deep venous thrombosis in the
        B   **True**   puerperium is increased threefold by forceps
        C   **False**   delivery when compared to normal vaginal delivery,
        D   **False**   and fourfold by postpartum sterilisation. The risk is
        E   **True**   increased tenfold by caesarean section. Epidural
                        anaesthesia in labour or induction with intravenous
                        Syntocinon do not increase the risk of deep venous
                        thrombosis. Suppression of lactation with
                        oestrogens significantly increases the incidence of
                        deep venous thrombosis and therefore should no
                        longer be used.

3.168   A   **False**   Superficial thrombophlebitis occurs in about 1% of
        B   **False**   pregnancies. An area around the superficial vein in
        C   **False**   the leg becomes painful, tender, red and swollen.
        D   **True**   This is due to venous clotting in a varicose vein and
        E   **False**   although called thrombophlebitis the condition is
                        one of inflammation not infection. There is no
                        hazard to the patient unless there is spread to deep
                        veins which is uncommon. Treatment is by
                        elevation and support of the affected part with mild
                        analgesics. Anticoagulation and antibiotics do not
                        help.

3.169   A   **False**   The majority of cases of deep vein thrombosis are
        B   **True**   either unrecognised or are treated adequately
        C   **True**   without further sequelae. When pulmonary
        D   **True**   embolism does occur, in over 50% of cases
        E   **False**   thrombosis elsewhere has not been recognised.
                        Although it usually presents as chest pain,
                        dyspnoea or haemoptysis, occasionally the first
                        sign may be the patient collapsing. It is now a
                        major cause of maternal death in the UK. Treatment
                        should always include anticoagulation.

3.170   A   **False**   The maternity or fourth day blues occur in up to
        B   **False**   50% of patients. The cause is uncertain, possibly
        C   **False**   hormonal changes, personality changes or the
        D   **False**   reaction to a major life event. There is no evidence
        E   **False**   for the condition being metabolic or
                        endocrinological. The patients are transiently tearful
                        and mildly depressed. Treatment involves support,
                        and anxiolytics are not necessary. Spontaneous
                        recovery is usual within 48 hours.

3.171 Postnatal depression
A   occurs in about 10% of women following delivery
B   usually occurs about 3–4 weeks following delivery
C   is increased in previously infertile women
D   if severe should be treated with tricyclic antidepressants
E   is a contraindication to breast feeding

3.172 Puerperal psychosis
A   occurs in about 2% of women
B   usually occurs about six weeks following delivery
C   is usually a manic affective disorder
D   is best treated in a mother and baby psychiatric unit
E   is very unlikely to occur in subsequent pregnancies

3.173 Postpartum sterilisation
A   should be performed laparoscopically
B   has a higher failure rate than sterilisation performed as an interval procedure
C   cannot be performed using Filshie clips
D   is the method of choice for women wishing sterilisation following delivery
E   has a higher 'regret rate' than an interval sterilisation

(Answers overleaf)

3.171 A **True**   Postnatal depression occurs in 10–15% of women
      B **False**   usually presenting between six and 12 weeks after
      C **True**   delivery. It is related to increasing maternal age,
      D **True**   previous subfertility, marital conflict, unwanted
      E **False**   pregnancy, unsatisfactory home support and
                    previous psychiatric problems. Most cases are of
                    moderate severity and treatment can be just
                    supportive. In severe cases treatment should be
                    with tricyclic antidepressant drugs. There is no
                    contraindication to breast feeding regardless of
                    whether the woman has been treated with tricylic
                    antidepressants or not.

3.172 A **False**   Puerperal psychosis occurs in about 1 in 500
      B **False**   pregnancies usually within 2–4 weeks of delivery. It
      C **False**   is usually a depressive affective disorder and mania
      D **True**   occurs only rarely. It is a serious condition and
      E **False**   need referral to a psychiatrist and treatment in a
                    mother and baby unit if one is available. The exact
                    treatment depends upon the type of psychosis. The
                    prognosis is good, most women leaving hospital
                    after two months. There is a recurrence risk of
                    5–10% in subsequent pregnancies and 30% go on
                    to develop psychotic conditions unrelated to
                    pregnancy.

3.173 A **False**   Postpartum sterilisation is usually performed 2–3
      B **True**   days following delivery compared with an interval
      C **False**   sterilisation which is usually performed six weeks
      D **False**   to three months following delivery. In the
      E **True**   puerperium the uterus is enlarged making
                    laparoscopy more dangerous. A postpartum
                    sterilisation should therefore be performed by a
                    mini-laparotomy. The tubes are thicker and more
                    vascular and the failure rate is 2–3 times higher
                    than that of sterilisation not performed in the
                    puerperium. Although the tubes are larger the
                    sterilisation can be performed with Filshie clips or
                    as a modified Pomeroy technique. Most women
                    who wish sterilisation following delivery should
                    have an interval procedure as the failure rate is
                    higher, the incidence of complication of, e.g. DVT, is
                    higher and the regret rate is higher with a
                    postpartum sterilisation.

3.174 The six week postnatal assessment
    A   is usually performed by the district midwife
    B   should include a haemoglobin estimation
    C   is not a good time to perform a cervical smear
    D   is the correct time to insert an IUCD if the patient wishes
         this for contraception
    E   should be performed before sexual intercourse is resumed

3.175 In the puerperium the community midwife
    A   will visit daily for the first three weeks
    B   will prescribe the oral contraceptive pill if required
    C   will palpate the abdomen
    D   will remove perineal sutures only under supervision by
         the GP
    E   is a significant source of psychological support for the
         mother

(Answers overleaf)

3.174 A **False**   The six week postnatal assessment is usually
      B **True**   performed by the general practitioner but in
      C **False**   complicated cases may be performed in the
      D **True**   hospital postnatal clinic. It should include a
      E **False**   haemoglobin estimation, weight, blood pressure,
urine analysis and cervical smear if indicated.
Sexual intercourse can be resumed at any time the
couple feel comfortable. The six week check is the
correct time to fit an IUCD as the uterus should
have returned to normal size by this time.

3.175 A **False**   The vast majority of puerperal care is provided by
      B **False**   the community midwife in a normal pregnancy.
      C **True**   This care will include palpation of the fundal height
      D **False**   and care of the perineum including removal of
      E **True**   sutures. They form the main source of professional
and psychological support during the puerperium
and although their remit includes contraceptive
advice they are unable to prescribe.

4. Bibliography

A discussion of the answers to these questions will be found in:

de Swiet M, Chamberlain G V P 1992 Basic Sciences in obstetrics and gynaecology, 2nd ed. Churchill Livingstone, Edinburgh
Elder M G 1988 Reproduction, obstetrics and gynaecology. Heinneman Medical Books, Oxford
Lewis T L T, Chamberlain G V P 1990 Obstetrics by 10 teachers, 15th ed. Edward Arnold, London
Shaw R W, Soutter W P, Stanton S L (eds) 1992 Gynaecology. Churchill Livingstone, Edinburgh
Symonds E M 1992 Essential obstetrics and gynaecology, 2nd ed. Churchill Livingstone, Edinburgh